Yoga of the Subtle Body

YOGA

of the Subtle Body

A Guide to the Physical and
Energetic Anatomy of Yoga

Tias Little

SHAMBHALA
Boulder
2016

Shambhala Publications, Inc.
2129 13th Street
Boulder, Colorado 80302
www.shambhala.com

14 13 12 11 10 9 8 7

Printed in United States of America

♾ This edition is printed on acid-free paper that meets the American National Standards Institute z39.48 Standard.
♻ Shambhala Publications makes every effort to print on recycled paper.
For more information please visit www.shambhala.com.

Shambhala Publications is distributed worldwide by Penguin Random House, Inc., and its subsidiaries.

Designed by Greta D. Sibley

Library of Congress Cataloging-in-Publication Data

Little, Tias, author.
Yoga of the subtle body: a guide to the physical and energetic anatomy of yoga / Tias Little.
Pages cm
ISBN 978-1-61180-102-6 (paperback)
1. Chakras. 2. Hatha yoga. I. Title.
BL1215.C45L58 2015
613.7'046—dc23
2013046152

Contents

Foreword

I extol bhavānī *whose body is nectar and whose very form is joy.*
She triumphantly shines forth at the end of a string of six lotuses.
Exceedingly lustrous in the middle way of the suṣumnā,
She melts the moon of nectar to drink its light.

—*Bhavāni Bhujaṅgam* of Śaṅkarācarya, verse 1[1]

The subtle body in yoga is not only the secret to the optimal functioning and alignment of the body; it is the key to delight, love, understanding, and good relationships. And subtle this body is! At times it dissolves into pure awareness and at other times it cranks out the endless fabric of daily life. The subtle body is often represented as being populated with gods, goddesses, wheels, flowers, amazing animals, and mythological realms. It maps the nature of mind and reality with its paradoxical loops and bright seas of nectar. We must constantly remember that *subtle* means mysterious, irreducible, delicate, and fine. Looking into subtle things tends to temporarily suspend the thinking process into a state of open inquiry and wonder.

We all have a subtle body, because we all have a body and a mind. Our minds make all kinds of images, symbols, and tags to remember, recognize, and organize experience. We plant those in the otherwise open, radiant, and unbiased tree of the sense fields. We push and pull on these symbols, tags, and ideas for they represent and map our vital interests, needs, hopes, and fears. Even when we think about subtle things like consciousness, God, or time, our minds create a symbolic representation for them all and arrange them like objects in various relationships. Because of this seemingly ceaseless symbol-making power of the mind, our experiences and our ideas about ourselves and others can be quite imbalanced, biased, and miserable. To be honest our subtle body is at least a little miserable most of the time. This misery that the subtle body suffers is caused by an ignorance in our minds that confuses the symbol with the thing or the map with the territory, while at the same time the mind tries in vain to make the subtle gross, the impermanent permanent, and the deep shallow.

The yoga and tantra traditions of India, Tibet, and Asia are happy to turn the mind back around on itself and contemplate the interfacing of myths, metaphors, and symbols with the everyday particulars of the breath and the experience of raw bodily sensation. Mindful awareness of internal breath and associated sensations and thoughts naturally reveals context, depth, and counterbalance to any mistakes of our mapping habits. Traditional yoga practices can speed up or encourage this process by having us visualize and feel areas of internal breath using colorful imagery, or reciting and directing *mantra* into specific places in or around the body. This allows us to experience things on a truly subtle level where labels and referential ideas temporarily fall away and the fullness of the interconnected world shines forth. Mind, thought, and image are used together to see through the overlapping confusions in those very thought processes. Subtle body meditation can eliminate the misperceptions that create suffering and confusion in the first place. As the subtle body is balanced and its channels opened free of bias, experiences come where each particular thing, thought, or sensation already contains all of the others, even to the point where each pore of the skin might contain a delightful universe, and each sensation point reveals delightful nectar. Ultimately the subtle body, your body, is meditated upon as the sacred, astonishing, and infinite body of pure awareness, intelligence, and compassion.

The beauty of Tias Little's book *Yoga of the Subtle Body* is that he delights in keeping the subtlety and mystery of the mind and the body. This keeps our minds open, so we continue to look, explore, and enjoy the fresh and always new face of reality. How exciting to explore with Little the detailed nature of anatomy, physiology, and neuroscience in relation to the ancient wisdom of yoga, the chakras, and *nāḍīs*. This grounding of the esoteric and the profound in the nitty-gritty of the body serves to sharpen the cutting edge of any yoga practice.

—Richard Freeman, Author of *The Mirror of Yoga*

Introduction

What is the subtle body? Is it something material like connective tissue, hormonal secretion, or neuronal pulse? Or is it formless, like space, pure energy, or consciousness? Is it tied to emotions such as fear or passion? In the tradition of yoga, the subtle body suggests that which is fine, delicate, and infinitesimally small such as an atomic particle. It also speaks to the all-pervading spirit in the body and is one of the names of Śiva.

In this book I undertake an investigation of the subtle body, bringing together notions of the animating spirit that appear in traditional yoga sources with the anatomical body. I will proceed to look at the body through a variety of different lenses—including the body as it is portrayed in classical Indian mythology, the esoteric anatomy of the chakra and *nāḍī* systems, and the structural body as it is charted in contemporary systems of holistic health.

While there are many books on yoga philosophy and also many books on anatomy, there are few that weave the two together. The intersection of mystical anatomy described in many old yoga texts with the body's glands, connective tissues, and organs has long been an interest of mine. My intention for this book is to provide insights into metaphysical speculations as they relate to the body, and through guided exercises, meditations, and reflections to give readers an experience of the subtle body.

When imagining the subtle body, the mystics and yogis of India and Tibet designed elaborate systems for navigating the body's interior, akin to the network circuitry of a computer. These systems map the flow of breath called *prāṇa* whose dynamic potency pumps, flows, and trickles through myriad channels, called *nāḍīs*. The exact nature of these pathways is difficult to articulate in any one biological system; their potency suggests a physio-spiritual force that transcends scientific rationale.

The language and imagery used to articulate the subtle body, in collections such as the Upaniṣads that date back as far as the fifth century B.C.E. and the *Haṭha Yoga Pradīpikā* in the fifteenth century C.E., are metaphorical and cryptic. This is due in part to the fact that the landscape of the inner body, long before the era of the microscope or magnetic resonance imaging (MRI), was visualized during states of profound meditation. Also descriptions of the subtle body were shrouded in metaphor and obscure so as not to be readily understood by the uninitiated but reserved for those who trained with a qualified master. Ironically, today we have the opposite scenario, where yoga teachings are ubiquitous, launched on the World Wide Web, and made available to everyone at any time.

In this book I attempt to capture some of the flavor of this metaphorical body and relate it to yoga practices today. This stems in part because as a teacher, I am drawn to the poetic imagination and use metaphor regularly when I teach. I believe that ultimately it is impossible to articulate the yogic experience in words. By articulating the body-mind connection through analogy and image (such as lifting the brain stem upward like the hood of a cobra), a direct experience of the subtle body becomes more palpable. Metaphorical thinking allows for greater flexibility, imagination, and openness, all of which are integral to the mind in meditation.

In writing this book, it became clear to me that in the eyes of the ancient seers of India, the form of the body is not simply utilitarian, whose purpose is to eat, sleep, and reproduce. Rather the body is a microcosmos where energies get played out. In it, sunlight is reflected, wind roams, rivers flow, and flowers bloom. It is where lotuses, turtles, serpents, and dragons dwell. In this sense the body is not to be taken literally but figuratively. Thus, in the history of yogic thought and practice, the subtle body not only involves complex and compelling biological rhythms but is the home of a multitude of archetypal forces.

Also, within the visual corpus of yoga-inspired art, the psychospiritual life has been rendered in wild and provocative ways. Through myth, sculpture, and story, benevolent and malevolent forces are carried out by multiheaded deities, treacherous demons, intricate mandalas, and animal spirits. For instance, Śiva, the arch yogi, is depicted riding a bull, seated atop the highest Himalayan peak (in the full lotus posture), in the form of a stone phallus (the *liṅga*), or as an androgynous being. In the art of yoga, the complexity of the human psyche gets expressed in ways that are at once multidimensional in form and affective singular in spirit.

The archetypal forces in the body are sustained by the vivifying effect of prāṇa. Prāṇa is a mysterious energy, the immeasurable source of life itself. As an avid practitioner and student of the internal arts, I have found it invaluable to understand the structures of the body through which this vivifying force of prāṇa flows. My studies began with how the musculoskeletal system relates to yoga postures and has evolved to include an understanding of how yoga practice affects digestion, circulation, and the flow of lymph and hormonal secretions. In this book on the subtle body, I detail how the anatomical architecture of the body provides organization and support for the flow of prāṇa through blood vessels, nerve tracts, and lymph capillaries. Prāṇa within the subtle body is impacted by the powerful effects of emotion. Thus, my research includes how divisive psychological and emotional states become embedded in the tissues of the body: buried under the skin, held in the pelvis, stuck in the diaphragm, or locked in the jaw.

Since the effects of stress and trauma, so prevalent in our world today, can disrupt the body's delicate balance dramatically, I dedicate time to discuss the effects of trauma on the subtle body. I then provide postures and meditations that help counter the effects of stress. In today's anxiety-ridden society, it is difficult to become what one of my meditation teachers described as a "happy, healthy human being." By looking closely at how psychosomatic stress today affects digestion, heart rate, sleep patterns, and musculoskeletal strain, I offer contemporary insights into an ancient tradition.

While it is valuable to study and reflect on the various systems of the body as unique (musculoskeletal, digestive, neurological, etc.), in a living being every structure in the body is interdependent. All connective tissue, every organ, every blood vessel, and every cell is interconnected within the body's overall fluid matrix. The notion of interdependency plays an important and powerful role in Hindu and Buddhist mythology. For instance, the well-known parable the Net of Indra depicts the interconnectivity of all phenomena, from the outermost corners of the galaxies and intergalactic dust to the cellular structure of the spleen and stomach. In the telling of the myth, the primeval god Indra has hung a vast net, one that extends infinitely in all directions. At each node in the net there is a perfectly clear gem that reflects all other gems in the net, so that the process of inter-reflection goes on and on. In this book I suggest that the body is a similar net, web, or continuum of interrelated structures. Understanding the interconnectivity of living structure leads to a more direct sensory experience of totality and integration on the mat.

The organization of the book follows an outline I have used in my yoga teacher trainings for over fifteen years. I follow a course upward through the body from the feet and legs, along the spine and trunk, to the crown of the head. By starting at the ground, the root, I travel from lower chakras to upper chakras, from coarse to subtle, and from dark to light. This follows a well-established trajectory in classical yoga that involves a passage from dormancy and inertia to illumined realization. I also point out how a series of horizontal structures in the body, here referred to as *diaphragms* (in the feet, pelvic floor, respiratory center, vocal cords, palate, and tentorium cerebelli), serve to orient posture and provide internal support.

In yoga today, the chakras are the most recognized representation of the subtle body. The word *chakra,* like many words in the Sanskrit language, has multiple meanings. It can mean a winding river, a cycle of years, a snake, a circular flight of birds, a potter's wheel, a prayer wheel, or an astronomical circle like the zodiac. In the body, the chakras are part of the imagined body: they have associations with geometric designs, animals, acoustic resonance, and are likened to blooming flowers. In the following chapters, I look at the metaphorical implication of each chakra along with its biological associations.

In keeping with the theme of the body as a relational field of interdependent structures and in keeping with the way our bipedal posture is organized from the ground up, I imagine the chakras beginning in the feet. Given the importance of the feet in helping align and stabilize the framework of the body, I decided to devote an entire chapter to the feet. In the sacred architecture of the body, the feet are the foundation to the temple. The feet and legs have important skeletal, fascial, and neurological connections to the spine. While the chapters herein trace the trajectory of the traditional spinal chakras, I have allocated an entire chapter to the respiratory diaphragm given its preeminent position in the body. The two chakras typically noted in the cranium, the third-eye center (*ājñā chakra*) and the crown (*sahasrāra chakra*), I cover together in one chapter, "The Crown Jewel."

Within the subtle body, the spine is the axis mundi, the channel through which the *kuṇḍalinī,* the primary biological force, is believed to reside. The midline of the body is relevant to the spinal cord, limbic brain, and autonomic nervous system. The middle axis through the body is charged with a kind of magnetic force (*śakti*), and its life-bestowing power is celebrated throughout yoga. I map the spine relative to the subtle body and delineate how the central nervous system is dependent on the peripheral nervous system, governed by the arms and legs.

My approach to the subtle body is interdisciplinary, and I mention other modalities of healing in addition to yoga. The following work then is a tapestry made from my own study and practice over the last thirty years. My perspective on the body is also shaped by insights I have gained from the world of manual therapy—particularly the practice of massage, Rolfing, craniosacral therapy, osteopathic medicine, Feldenkrais Method, and Thomas Hanna Somatics.

While I guide readers to sensorimotor experiences of the subtle body, this is not a how-to yoga book. Learning yoga, like learning a foreign language, requires first-person contact and the watchful eye and guiding touch of a teacher. First and foremost, this book is meant to inspire students, connoisseurs, and beginners alike to look at structural alignment and the energy body in fresh and novel ways. As Marcel Proust wrote, "The real voyage of discovery consists not in seeing new landscapes, but seeing with new eyes." My intention is to enhance the reader's process of discovery, to introduce new pathways of awareness, and to inspire insight.

The greatest danger in yoga, that by necessity involves routine, is becoming mechanical and regimented. I find that the beauty of a mind-body discipline, such as yoga or qigong, is that it is an endless process of discovery and surprise. This is frequently overlooked by students, driven by gain and bent on mustering as much strength and flexibility as possible. I think that yoga, rather than a path leading to mastery, is an invitation to evoke mystery and channel a powerful, subtle, and ultimately unnameable energy that roams inside. A dedicated practice is like a rite of passage that guides one to sense, feel, and remember that which inevitably resists identification. I can testify that the further I travel into the inner processes of the body and mind, the more I realize I don't know. The following words of Ken Kesey speak to this process of discovery and the necessity to invoke mystery.

> The answer is never the answer. What's really interesting is the mystery. If you seek the mystery instead of the answer, you'll always be seeking. I've never seen anybody really find the answer—they think they have, so they stop thinking. But the job is to seek mystery, evoke mystery, plant a garden where

> strange plants grow and mysteries bloom. The need for mystery is greater than the need for an answer.[1]

Explorations within the subtle body are something like cultivating a garden "where strange plants grow and mysteries bloom." I trust that this book will help plant seeds for practitioners to experience deeper and more nuanced explorations of their innermost being. I have found that the real joy of discovery occurs in the multiple and intricate connections to be made in the body-mind, connections that ultimately provide a profound sense of wholeness and integration.

1

FROM THE GROUND UP

The Journey from Root to Crown

I honor the lotus feet of all the ancestral teachers,
Which awaken and manifest joy in oneself,
Beyond comparison, appearing as a snake-charmer (Śiva)
For pacifying the poisonous delusion of saṃsāra (the cycle of birth and death).[1]

—From the Aṣṭāṅga -Yoga Mantra

In the part of the world where I live, the Southwestern United States, there is a long history of native people making their home along the Rio Grande valley. In the belief system of the ancient Anasazi people who lived here, human beings originate from down inside the womb of the earth. The journey to the earth's surface, the trek upward to birth and life, was understood as the migration of the soul of the people. The myth of the origins of Native American Pueblo tribes has remarkable similarities to the journey through the spinal centers within the yogic system. Themes of transformation abound, from dark to light, from inertia to enlivenment, from gross to subtle, and from depths to surface.

In Native American lore the earth is the mother, the progenitor of all life. This is suggested by the kiva ceremony (kivas are sacred, womblike subterranean spaces) where shamans, seers, and Pueblo folk descend down a wood-framed ladder, to pray, reflect, and commune. The myth that the earth is the origin of life for the Anasazi people was retold during a seminar held in Vienna in 1932 on the psychology of kuṇḍalinī yoga presented by C. G. Jung. Jung compared the Native American creation myth to progression through the chakras, which begin in the pelvic basin within the earthbound *mūlādhāra chakra* and continue to the crown of the head where, as celebrated in various invocations to the sage Patañjali, a "thousand heads of white light" radiate.

> There is a Pueblo myth [in] which man was generated far down in the earth in a pitch-black cave . . . After a dormant and absolutely dark worm-like existence, they found a cane which was like a ladder, so mankind could climb up and reach the floor of the next cave. Then they climbed up and reached the third cave . . . finally they came to the fourth cave. . . That cave opened out upon the earth . . . and they learned to make a brilliant light, out of which finally the sun and the moon were made.[2]

This is a tale of ascension from interior, subconscious, cavernous centers within the earth to creation, birth, and the rise of consciousness. We can think of elevation through the chakras in the same way. They involve stages of awakening, from the feet to the crown of the head. The chakras, like the caves in the Native American myth, are transitional places in the process of upward migration. In the Anasazi myth, the cane or ladder (the ladder is an archetype signifying psychological and spiritual transformation) is the means to climb. The plant used to ascend out of the depths in the Pueblo myth shares a likeness with the spinal cord, likened to a stalk or stem of a plant in the yoga tradition. This ladder resembles the central axis through the body that yogis consider to be the primary pathway that leads from the earthbound tailbone to the sky within the skull.

The earth is the beginning of the journey; it is the birthplace, the primal source, the womb from which all living things emerge and to which, in time, they return. Migration through the chakras begins underground, proceeds to the earth's surface, and advances on the vertical axis. Like a plant seedling breaking ground, like the bones of the body growing upward to stand, like the upright monoliths of Stonehenge, or the rising cobra, the human spirit evolves through vertical ascent.

PRACTICE

Śavāsana, the Ground Zero

Śavāsana, the corpse pose, is typically done at the end of a practice session; however, I frequently begin my classes with śavāsana, for it allows students to release their body, to empty themselves of muscular tension, and to drop, via gravity, into the earth. Śavāsana is a pose where the body is fully supported, resting horizontally, so that a profound stillness and quiescence can penetrate inside. Ultimately, letting go in śavāsana suggests not a physical death but a spiritual death (*mahā samādhi*) where all traces of a self limited by personal identity drop away and one experiences boundlessness and peace.

Begin by lying on your back on a soft but firm floor support. Exhale deeply several times and allow the weight of your bones to drop into the floor, and in turn, to the ground below the floor. Allow the weight of your organs to sink, like leaves lowering to the bottom of a winter pond. Visualize your blood and breath settling into the back of your body. Allow your skin to spread out along the floor, so that the skin of your back body is fully in contact with the floor. Allow the weight of the back of your sacrum and the weight at the back of your skull to drop. Inhale into your back ribs and feel them expand against the floor. Sense your prāṇic sheath (*prāṇa-maya-kośa*). Ask yourself, are you tired, bloated, restless, heavy, or distracted? Do you have any pain that is palpable? Scan your body for any nuance of sensation; that is, notice any tingle or pulsation in your nerves, bloodstream, or fascia. By developing sensitivity to the smallest of sensations, you will be able to attune to the subtle body. Stay for ten minutes before slowly rolling to your side to come out.

The Feet as Gateways to Transformation

For bipedal man the feet tread the dust of the earth, and throughout history walking on terra firma has involved migration and transformation—being on the move. In Native American cultures of the Southwest, tribal people would run for miles from one community to the next. In India and Tibet, pilgrimages to sacred geographic sites involve trekking for miles. In biblical lore, passage through the desert suggested an exodus, a migration away from the confines of both authoritarian power and a limited psyche. In the structure of the body, the plantar surface of the foot connects to the ground and thus is the genesis for evolution.

A disciplined journey through the labyrinthine channels of the subtle body—through bone, tissue, cells, and hormonal secretions—necessarily begins with the feet. In light of the itinerant, fast-paced, and highly mobile society we live in today, establishing a sense of ground through the feet is valuable. Generating stability and support through the bones and connective tissues of the feet can help regulate the nervous system, increase circulation, and improve respiration. The earthward rooting of the foundation of the body can help bring composure in the face of difficulty, whether it is a fragmented family, a health crisis, a failing marriage, or a precarious economy. To this end, standing poses in yoga help build endurance, steadiness, and resolve.

Earth, Primary within the Five Elements

In the internal arts of India, China, and Japan the body is thought to be a composite of elemental forces; that is, its bones, skin, and secretions are made of the same raw materials as the natural world. The chakras derive from the elements that are associated with each bodily center and the feet are associated with the base element of earth.[3] Celebratory passages from the *Taittirīya Upaniṣad* imagine a successive origination of matter from pure consciousness down to the solidity of earth associated with the feet and pelvis:

> From the ātman manifests space, from space air, from air fire, from fire water, from water earth, from earth the plants, from plants food, and from food humankind.[4]
>
> Throughout this exploration of the subtle body, we will refer to the physiology of the five elements as they correlate to the spine, internal organs, and the endocrine glands (fig. 1.1).

This chapter examines how the feet are the foundation for the temple of the body. The challenge of a yoga practice is similar to the challenge faced by a builder or engineer: the first task is to set the foundation. Structurally, the feet support the body and are the source for numerous nāḍīs and meridian channels. The soles of the feet underpin all bodily systems, so that posturally, all weight-bearing forces are borne by the feet. Arrangement of the twenty-six bones in the feet

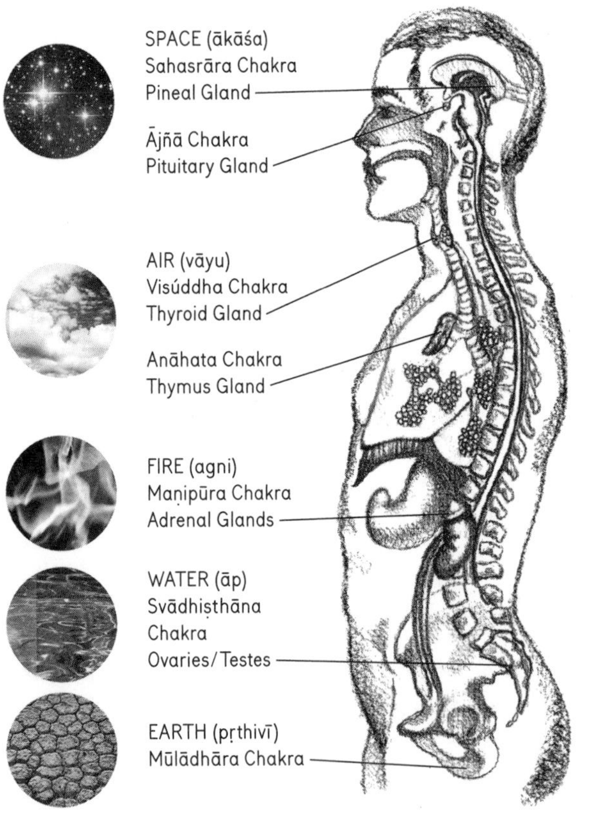

Figure 1.1 The Subtle Body: Chakras, Glands, and the Five Elements

determine, to a large degree, balance in all higher structures. Aberrations in the ankles and feet translate to twists, torques, and rotations above. Given that the feet stand under the entire body, we will see how it is critical to *understand* the dynamics of the feet. The first challenge in yoga is to relearn how to stand.

Feet as Tree Roots

Developing the *mind* of the feet is an important part of training in the internal arts. One of the first challenges of a yoga teacher is to encourage his or her students to bring wakefulness and structural integrity to the small bones and ligaments of their feet—the taproots of their body. That the body is like a tree is one of the oldest analogies in yoga. In the tree metaphor, the toes and feet nourish the body in the same way that the roots of a tree draw water, nutrients, and minerals out of the ground in order to support the vitality of the trunk, branches, and leaves. In turn, the spine supports the growth of the arms and hands like a tree trunk supports the branches and leaves. Ultimately the roots of the feet help metabolize prāṇa by remotely providing support to fine twiglike structures within the lungs (bronchioles) together with their alveoli leaf clusters.

The multiple small bones of the feet help distribute and support the weight of the entire frame adequately at the base of the body. A network of numerous small ligaments and muscles anchor the bones of the feet like the prolific roots of a banyan tree. The multiple tendons and ligaments provide stability and malleability in the feet during standing, walking, and running.

By establishing an extensive root system through the feet—stretching the plantar fascia, spreading the metatarsal bones, broadening the heel, and lifting the arches of the feet—we provide structural organization for the entire body.

Tree Pose

Of all yoga poses *vṛkṣāsana*, the tree pose, is the quintessential position for gaining concentrated powers of attention. To gain *tapas* or spiritual vitality, yogis have been known to stand in tree pose for months and even years. *Taḍāsana* (mountain pose) has a similar significance. In B. K. S. Iyengar's seminal text on yoga postures, *Light on Yoga,* taḍāsana and vrksāsana are the first two poses.

One example of the key historical significance of tree pose is depicted in the Descent of the Ganges, a ninety-six-foot-long narrative carved into a monolithic boulder. Located in Mahabalipuram in South India and a World Heritage Site, the massive rock relief was created in the mid-seventh century; its cosmological scene relates the origin of life. Multiple figures surround the downward flow of the river Ganga (featured as a natural cleft in the rock and reminiscent of the central channel of the body) and at the source of the life-bestowing river stands a yogi in tree pose. The carved ascetic, a gaunt figure with protruding ribs, gives the illusion that he is holding up the mountain, so that the mother of all rivers, the sacred Ganga, can flow unobstructed. In yoga, we can think of tree pose, given its antiquity and simple power, upholding the entire haṭha yoga tradition.

Structure of the Foot

We now turn our attention to the architecture of the foot that serves as a blueprint for the entire body.

The Sole of the Foot

The sole of the foot is the first horizontal diaphragm in the body; it hugs the earth, melding to the contour of the ground. More than thirty joints within the foot make continuous micro-adjustments while you're walking and standing. The fact that there is one bone in the upper leg (the femur), two in the lower leg (the tibia and fibula), and twenty-six in the feet indicates the degree of potential articulation within the foot. Yet the full range of motion within the foot typically goes underutilized. For many people, the complex network of tissues in the foot contort, constrict, and harden. As we construct the temple of the body from the ground up, the location of the plantar surface of the foot—right at ground level—is indispensable for laying a firm foundation.

There is little padding and no musculature on the superior surface of the foot. If you palpate the top of your foot, you will feel the long, ropy tendons that transit downward from the tibia and fibula and track across the long bones of your feet (metatarsals). However, the sole of the foot is composed of a half-inch-thick pad. For this reason, support for the foot comes not only from the long guy-wire tendons that suspend the foot from the shin bones but from a bed of muscles and tendons four layers thick at the sole of the foot.

The plantar fascia, the superficial layer of this bed of muscles and tendons on the underside of the foot, is a strong webbing that functions like a snowshoe; it is elastic, resilient, and tough, enabling the long metatarsal bones to spring off the floor. This ropy, tensile webbing attaches to the heel and to the roots of all five toes. Behind the tendinous girder of the plantar fascia are multiple short muscles that control fine articulations within the foot.

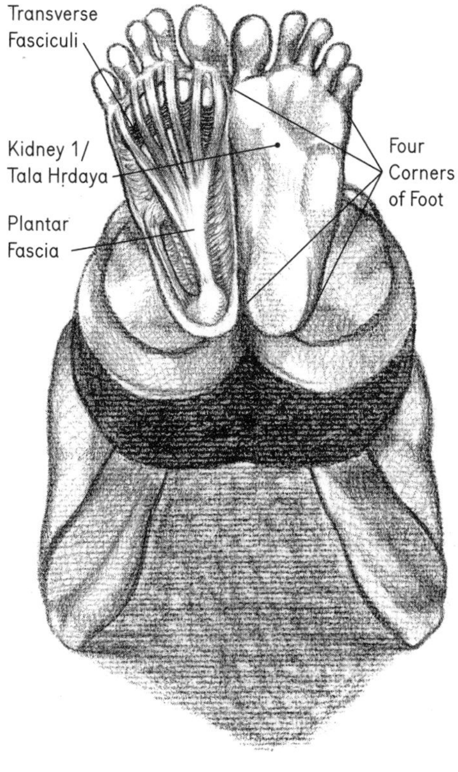

Figure 1.2 The First Diaphragm: Plantar Fascia Shown in Shoulder Stand

The plantar fascia continues via a sinewy fascial stocking over the heel (calcaneus), whereupon it weaves into the Achilles tendon. Together the plantar fascia and Achilles tendon form a robust sling, one that is in constant demand to hold the body upright and stable. There are a number of activities that causes this sling to become taut and inflexible; standing for long hours, running or walking long distances on pavement, and wearing unsupportive footwear. One of the common postural patterns that causes the Achilles plantar–tendon fascia sling to tighten is a stance that involves a forward thrust of the leg. When the femur and tibia lurch forward, this sling at the base of the dorsal leg (the back leg) locks long. Like a tree trunk that pitches forward and must be propped upright by a landscaper's supporting cables, a forward-thrusting leg is held upright by the plantar fascia–Achilles tendon sling. Rigidity in the plantar fascia–Achilles tendon sling is a common barrier to progress in yoga; it will cause inflexibility in the foot and calf, thus limiting a yoga student's ability to squat with her heels on the floor or ground her heels in *adho mukha śvānāsana* (downward-facing dog pose).

Activating the multiple ligaments, tendons, and bones of the foot is critical in all poses—standing poses, forward bends, backbends, and seated poses. It is also important to extend out through the feet in inversions such as *śirṣāsana* (headstand) or *sarvāṅgāsana* (shoulderstand). If the feet are dead weight in inverted positions, then the neck, skull, or shoulders may suffer from compression. A well-performed inversion is like an upside-down standing pose as the plantar fascia of the foot is actively stretched and lengthened (fig. 1.2). Not only do the soles of the feet provide structural support; they also help "fuel" the leg. When inverted, the feet perform like solar panels; they are conductors of kinetic energy, and so we could think of them collecting and distributing prāṇa throughout the body. This is also the case when walking or standing barefoot on the beach or ground—the soles of the feet absorb the earth's magnetic field and negative ions, thought to boost biochemical activity in the body, increase levels of mood-enhancing serotonin, and relieve stress.

Arches and Bridges in the Foot

The design of the foot includes arches and bridges that provide support for the entire body. Yoga practice is always done barefoot, as the barefooted position affords greater connection to the ground and helps to gird up the arches of the feet.

There are three arches within the foot—medial, lateral, and transverse. Of the three, the medial arch is the most critical as it affords connection to the core and provides support for the inside leg, inner groin muscles, and pelvic floor. Furthermore, raising the inner foot arch gives access to the delicate structures of the spinal chakras within the subtle body. Lift of the medial arch involves elevating the inner ankle bone (base of the tibia) and raising a bone called the navicular. The navicular bone is the keystone of the inner arch.

The lateral arch involves lift of the outer edge of the foot and the lateral ankle (the base of the fibula). The lateral arch provides stability for the outer leg including the outer knee, iliotibial band, and outer hip. The keystone to the lateral arch is the cuboid bone, a stout, square bone that articulates with the navicular. Together they form a sturdy strut right through the heart of the foot. The transverse arch, the third arch, spans across the bones of the feet and provides a domelike contour to the bones of the midfoot. The three arches function like a trampoline in that they provide spring and suspension. In the design of the trampoline, the powerful springs that anchor the taut nylon webbing to its border are like the resilient ligaments and tendons that hold the bones of the foot together.

The span between the base of the little toe and the base of the big toe is like a miniature bridge. The bases of the first and fifth metatarsals are cornerstones to this bridge and are the primary pressure points for weight bearing. (If you look at the sole of your foot, you should see that they are more calloused, as they bear the load when standing and during the push-off phase of the gait.) By actively spreading the pedestals of the toes in standing positions, this metatarsal bridge gains greater stability and lift. When creating span across the bridge of the toes and foot, one stretches the small slips of connective tissue that form a horizontal webbing across the plantar fascia. (Notice in figure 1.2 the transverse fasciculi across the distal end of the plantar fascia.)

In a healthy and competent foot, there is span, height, and spring to these vital struts. In turn, the arches and bridges provide a lift for the frame of the entire body. Unfortunately, it is all too common for the beams, girders, and cables within the foot bridge to buckle, resulting in a downward sag. A collapsed foot has reduced resilience and spring, potentially causing compaction and concretion within the foot, ankles, and knees. As a result, the entire foot structure may have little give. Due to this inflexibility, balance becomes unsteady, shaky, and tottery. Good circulation and metabolic exchange in the lower limb may be compromised, excess fluid can accumulate, resulting in edema, varicose veins, or spider veins. One of the consequences of fallen arches may be gripping or clenching in the musculature of the buttocks, hip joints, and lower back. Disorganization and spatial displacement in the ankle or foot may cause structures higher up to twist, rotate, or collapse.

When the bones of the feet and their surrounding tissues collapse, it feels like driving a vehicle with flat tires. The suspension system cannot sufficiently support the axle, struts, and frame. In this case, the frame caves, the vehicle has little capacity for shock absorption, and the car is prone to bottoming out. If the suspension system of the foot deflates, the lower back is made particularly vulnerable. If the feet and ankles collapse, then not only is the lower back vulnerable but overall vitality in the body can wane, and people are more prone to fatigue and exhaustion.

The Heel Strike

The heel, also called the calcaneus, is the hardest bone in the body. This is understandable given the heel's role in bearing the weight of the entire body in standing and walking. The plantar fascia attaches to the anterior heel. When the plantar fascia is tight, not only can it yank the heel forward, shortening the span of length between heel and toes, but it can pull away from the bone, causing bone spurs.

The heel bone has a peculiar spherical shape, and it is not a surprise that forces transmitted into the heel often carom to one side. This can cause the heel to either roll to the inside or pitch to the outside. How postural weight drops into the heel determines, in large part, how patterns of strain are held in the leg. When it comes to balancing the heel, standing poses are ideal for aligning the heels. In time this can alter how weight falls into the heel in walking, called the heel strike. Pressing into the heels in standing postures is a bit like playing billiards. The angle at which one presses the heel will determine the trajectory of forces that relay up the inside or outside leg, in turn affecting the inner or outer edges of the leg and pelvis.

When standing, we must ask: Am I collapsing to the inner or outer edge of my heel? One good way to assess heel strike and the distribution of weight into your heel is to examine an old favorite pair of boots or sneakers. Is the inner pad of the shoe heel worn down or the outer? How weight caroms to one side of the heel may translate to further collapsing higher up the leg.

PRACTICE

Trikonāsana, Śiva's Trident, and Finding the Center Heel

During standing positions in yoga, it is important to discern which part of the heel anchors to the floor—the inner, outer, or center heel. I imagine these three aspects of the heel to be like Śiva's trident, a three-pronged configuration that suggests a trinity (fig. 1.3). This trinity describes not only a dynamic play between inner-outer-center but other triads such as future-present-past and creation-preservation-destruction.

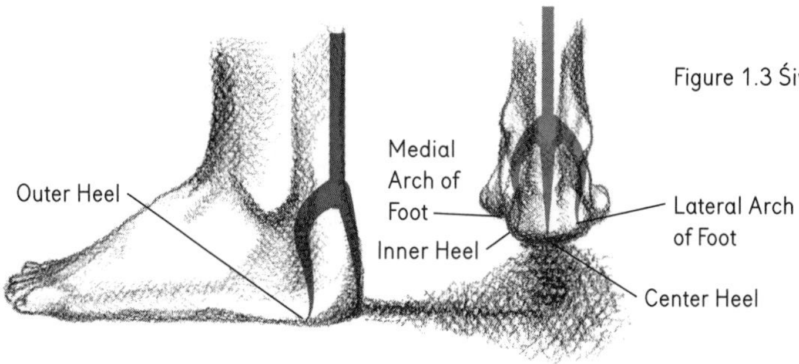

Figure 1.3 Śiva's Trident and the Heel Bone

For triangle pose, step your feet three to four feet apart. Turn your right foot out so that the inner edge of your right foot is parallel to the long side of your mat. Turn your back foot in twenty degrees. Look down and notice where your weight falls into your front heel. Typically the weight shears to the outside heel due to tension on the outside leg. Press down on your inside heel, pinning down the inner prong of the trident. At the same time elevate the inner arch of your front foot (including the navicular bone). Then notice the heel of your back leg. The weight typically collapses to the inside heel, given the weakness and collapse of the inside leg, so tack down the outer edge of your back heel (the outer fork of Śiva's trident). This movement is particularly important for people who have suffered lateral ankle sprains and have scar tissue built up in and around their outer ankle. Stretch your arms out and lengthen to your right into *trikonāsana.* Simultaneously press the inner prong of your front heel and the outer prong of your back heel down (without losing contact with the floor with the outer heel of your front foot and inner heel of your back foot). Stay for one minute, pull up to center, and switch sides.

After triangle pose, return to *samasthiti* (even standing) with your feet hip-width apart. Align your heels directly underneath your sitting bones. In your mind's eye map an imaginary trident, with prongs facing downward, onto your heels. Press the middle prong, your center heel, into the floor while lifting and spreading all ten toes. This center heel helps orient the midline of the leg, the center sitting bone, and the central spine.

PRACTICE

Anchoring the Four Corners of the Foot

Stand in tāḍāsana such that your feet are hip-width apart and press firmly into the base of your first metatarsal, the mound of your big toe. Imagine that you could impress the swirls of skin at the base of your big toe mound into your sticky mat so as to stamp a clear imprint. Then make contact with the little toe mound at the base of your fifth metatarsal and press. These are the front two corners of your foot (fig. 1.2). Be sure to spread the skin and connective tissue as much as possible between these two anchoring points both on the sole of your foot and the top of your foot. This serves to broaden the bridge that spans across the toes and make your toes more elastic.

Then tack down the inner edge of your heel and the outer edge of your heel simultaneously. These are the back two corners of the sole of your foot. Then press all four corners into the floor at the same time. In doing so, lift the bones, ligaments, and musculature of your foot matrix upward toward your knee. Then vault the four corners of your knee upward: the lower two corners below your kneecap, and upper two corners above your kneecap. This will increase the lift of your quadricep muscles and pump prāṇa back to your lungs. Continue to press into the four corners of your foot in order to build a firm foundation for your entire leg. Feel a current travelling upward through the bony shafts of your legs into your pelvis. Hold the pose for one to three minutes.

Activating the Medial Arch

Press down the ball mound of your big toe to spring-load the inner arch of your foot. Note that on the drawing of the lotus feet (fig 1.4), the big toe mound is rendered as a temple gate. Thus we could imagine how the first metatarsal not only is a significant bony landmark but serves as a doorway into the sanctum of the subtle body. Spread the webbing between your big toe and second toe. Press into the base of your big toe, leveraging your inside foot, inner knee, inner groins, and the front edge of your spine. Then, at the same time, press down through the outer edge of your heel. In your mind's eye, draw a diagonal across the sole of your foot by simultaneously pressing the base of your big toe and outer heel down. Feel the powerful lift of your inner ankle and inner arch this way.

Set a block on its face between the inner edges of both big toes. Keep your feet parallel and squeeze into the side of the block in order to elevate your two inner ankle bones. By pressing medially into the block (called adduction), you should feel your inner ankle bones vault upward. Avoid clenching or gripping your toes. Continue to spread your toes and press down into the ball mound of your big toe. Feel the way the entire inner channel of your leg engages, especially your inner knee and upper inner thigh. Hold for one to three minutes.

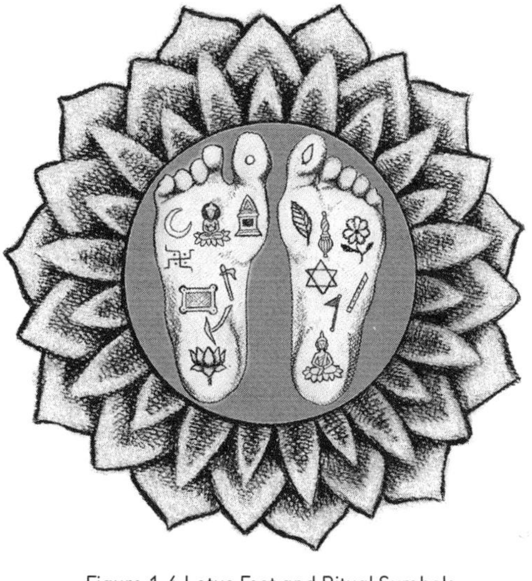

Figure 1.4 Lotus Feet and Ritual Symbols Related to the Subtle Body

Foot Reflexology: A Blueprint for the Body

Foot reflexology is a theoretical science that maps the body's organs, glands, and cavities onto the plantar surface of the foot (see fig. 1.5). It suggests that the entire body can be charted on the sole of the foot, such that the foot becomes a blueprint for the body's physical and organic structure. Various zones on the sole of the foot are thought to reflect different areas of the body, such as the lungs, kidneys, or large intestine. In yoga postures, forces applied to local regions of the foot generate referred movement into the pelvis, abdomen, neck, and head. For example, by extending the inner edge of the heel in a pose like half moon (ardha chandrāsana), one can achieve a corresponding move-

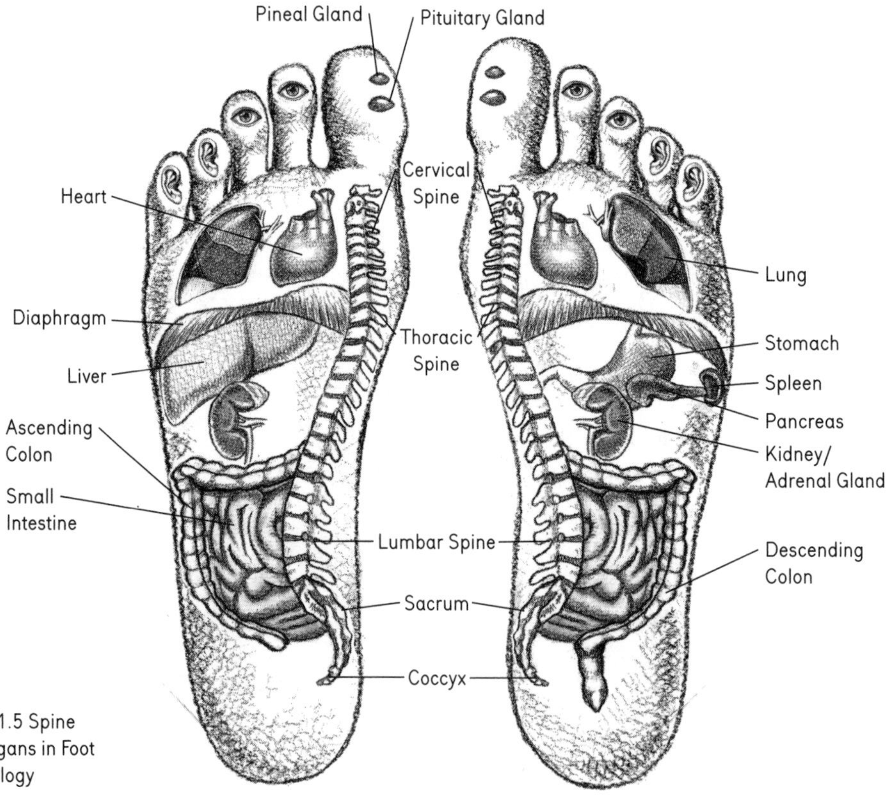

Figure 1.5 Spine and Organs in Foot Reflexology

ment in the tailbone area. (Notice the location of the coccyx on the inner heel in figure 1.5.) Movement of the inner heel thus remotely influences the bioenergetics of *mūlạ bandha*, the root lift of the pelvic diaphragm that we will explore in detail in the next chapter.

The Toes

The distal ends of the toes are like insect antennae. They help with postural balance, spatial orientation, and navigation. Yet as people age, the toes become stiff and rigid like wooden pegs. Toes become twisted and clenched and lose sensorimotor input. They lose agility and adaptability. Like loss of vision, inflexible toes make an elderly person prone to falling. Falling is one of the great nemeses of aging.

With this in mind, it is valuable for students to maintain or reestablish connection with their toes. A common cue a yoga teacher gives her students early in a practice is "spread your toes." There is a yoga prop designed to help passively spread the toes (it resembles the toe spreader used by pedicurists) that is a good tool to broaden the webbing between the metatarsals. In order to actively open the toes and webbing between the toes, I frequently teach what I call the broken-toe pose, a variation of *vajrāsana* or thunderbolt pose, described in detail on the next page. I have also taught classes in which I invite students to happily regress to the crawling stage to re-create somatic connection to their toes and foot arches, for the cross crawl is done with the toes and foot in flexion. In standing poses, it is crucial to articulate the toes by lifting and spreading them as if opening an oriental fan. In a pose like *ardha chandrāsana,* or half moon pose, this serves to activate the eye-toe reflex arc and to give the practitioner greater balance. Note in figure 1.5 how in foot reflexology the toe pads correlate to the eyes.

PRACTICE

Building the Dome of the Transverse Arch

This technique helps to build lift in the transverse arch of the foot. Begin by rolling up a thin sticky mat into a tight roll about two inches in circumference. For these two exercises be sure the roll is neither too bulky nor too puny. It should fit the contour of the sole of your foot. Stand facing a wall, at a distance where you can place your hands to the wall and thereby set your arms and trunk parallel to the floor. Place the sticky mat tube crosswise underneath the middle of both of your feet, so that the center of your foot contours over the tube. See that the four corners of your feet remain on the floor. In the wall dog position, actively stretch the long bones of your feet over the sticky mat tube. Observe the way that your transverse arch becomes concave below and convex above. Note the way that the long bones of your feet (metatarsals) spread both lengthwise and widthwise. Actively spread your toes in order to generate movement in the small bones of your feet. Observe any changes in your knees, femurs, and hips. Stay for one to three minutes, walk your hands up the wall, and step off of the sticky mat roll.

Then proceed to take the roll of your mat underneath the transverse arch of your front foot in triangle pose. Your foot should form a bridge over the roll. Press into your center heel (the middle fork of the trident) and base of your big toe and feel the way that the bones of your feet lift and spread. Stay for a minute before exiting and repeat on the other side. After doing both sides, stand in tāḍāsana in order to balance both feet and legs.

PRACTICE

Vajrāsana

Vajra in Sanskrit means "lightning," and for those with unyielding toes, this pose can feel like a fiery bolt. Begin in *bālāsana* (child's pose) and set your feet in flexion so your toes turn under. Extend your arms out in front of you, press your hands to the floor, and drive the weight of your sitting bones toward your heels. Stay for a minute. Then keep your feet in flexion and come to an upright kneeling position. If the load on your flexed toes is overwhelming, remain with your hands on the floor, come partially upright, and use your hands to adjust how much weight stacks onto the base of your toes. Another option to relieve the pressure in vajrāsana is to set a block between your heels and your buttocks.

Be sure that your toes are spread and your feet are just two to three inches apart. Can the base of your big toe make contact with the floor? Which big toe mound is less pliable? In time the toes and the long bones of your feet form a right angle. Interlock your fingers, extend your arms in front of your chest, and with your palms facing away from you, raise your arms. This is *baddha hastāsana* (bound hand pose) in vajrāsana. Draw the sides of your waist upward and lift the skin and flesh below your navel, as in *uḍḍīyāna bandha*. (For a description of uḍḍīyāna bandha, see page 118.) Stay for thirty seconds to a minute. In order to come out of the pose, lower your arms, point your toes back, and release back to child's pose.

As Below, So Above

Distortion and asymmetry accumulate in the feet, ankles, and lower limbs as we age. Many people have unequal leg lengths, and most people do not stand symmetrically or walk straight. Due to repetitive strain, trauma, or poor postural habits, asymmetries may develop: one leg may be longer than the other, one knee more rotated, the arch of one foot more collapsed. It is valuable for students of movement to come to *read* which foot is more stable and which is more prone to collapse. For movement therapists, analyzing the structures of the lower limbs—the orientation of the knee, shape of the fibularis muscles, tone of the gastrocnemius muscle, integrity of the foot arches—is critical for assessing the competency of the client's overall structure and the efficiency of her gait. In this sense, we follow the maxim *as below, so above.*

It takes considerably more physical energy to compensate for a misaligned structure than to maintain a structure that is balanced. When there is distortion, shearing, pulling, or collapse in one area of the body (in particular in the feet and legs), other neighboring structures are solicited to engage. Sustaining compensatory muscular holding takes energy just as an afflictive behavioral pattern in a dysfunctional relationship eats up available emotional (and physical) resources. Thus, if a series of postural holding patterns develop, it can literally be a drag. Moshe Feldenkrais, in *Body and Mature Behavior,* wrote,

> When its centre of gravity is maintained at the highest possible position, the human body is fit to move in any direction

> with practically no expenditure of energy, and even this minimum is drawn from its potential energy. The potential energy is restored afterwards so that all movement starts from this configuration of maximum potential energy.[5]

All mind-body disciplines within the internal arts aim to cultivate this "highest possible position" that minimizes energy expenditure. En route to this, it is important to identify compensatory patterns in the feet, knees, and pelvis and then apply techniques that are most appropriate to balance and reorganize. Via structural rebalancing, the body is imbued with optimal vitality and stamina.

Standing Poses

In practices such as yoga, tai chi, and qigong, standing positions aim to establish width, strength, span, and adaptability within the feet. Tāḍāsana, the first position in yoga, best embodies this integration. For instance in the methodology of Aṣṭāṅga Vinyāsa Yoga, a system that I trained in for fifteen years, practitioners return to tāḍāsana after each pose. In this way, one always returns to center, to the configuration of maximum potential energy.

Via the standing poses, students begin to release tightness and congestion in their feet. One culprit that is a common cause of clenching and constriction in the feet is footwear. Athletic cleats, ballet slippers, rock climbing shoes, work boots, and high heels potentially confine and constrict. By spreading the toes in yoga postures and lifting the foot arches and bridges, kinetic energy can circulate more efficiently through the entire body. In both the Aṣṭāṅga Vinyāsa and Iyengar Yoga systems, standing poses are the cornerstones of the practice. They are taught prior to seated poses, backbends, or inversions.

In particular, one-legged standing balance poses, such as tree pose or half moon pose, develop integrity and proficiency in the ligaments, tendons, and musculature surrounding the ankles and feet.

Mountain Pose

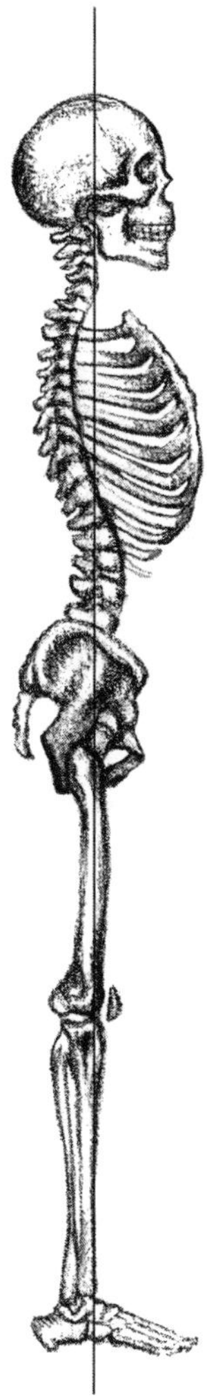

Figure 1.6
Plumb Line
Tāḍāsana

As noted earlier, the very first position in yoga is called tāḍāsana (mountain pose). To stand in tāḍāsana is to stand with ease, resolve, adaptability, and grace. Mountain pose is the first of all the standing positions and in many respects is the blueprint for all the āsanas—inversions, backbends, twists, and forward bends. In tāḍāsana, we stand in the sacred midline of the body (see fig. 1.6). In the meditative arts, the mountain is not limited to a postural stance but suggests the embodiment of wisdom.

The mountain implies not simply a static, unchanging block but a living, evolving, dynamic thing. In Zen training, the body is a mountain that walks, a concept enacted daily in group walking meditation (called *kinhin*). To embody the mountain suggests unalterable firmness and resolve on one hand and fluidity, impermanence, and change on the other. Zen master Dogen, founder of the Soto school of Japanese Buddhism in the year 1240, composed the "Mountains and Water Sutra" in which he describes mountains as the "bones and marrow of the Buddha ancestors." He describes "mountains as the realm where all buddhas practice" and "embody buddha's inconceivable qualities."[6]

In yoga, tāḍāsana may also be called samasthiti, which suggests "even standing" or the "stand of equanimity." *Sama,* like the English word *same,* suggests equality, congruency, and poise. The Sanskrit verbal root *stha* means to stand, take place, and have stability. Thus, the pose samasthiti implies balancing in graceful equilibrium on the plumb line of the body.

Learning to Stand on Both Feet

I recall a class I taught several years back for eighth graders at a local middle school in Santa Fe. One of the poses I had them do was tāḍāsana, and I was amazed to see how much of a challenge it was for fourteen-year-olds to stand upright without collapse. The kids fought the impulse to slouch, roll to the outside of their feet, cave in their chest, or pitch their head to one side. The seemingly simple act of standing upright, like a mountain, was foreign to them. Learning to stand on both feet is a valuable exercise to establish a sense of grounded awareness, centeredness, and personal self-worth at any age.

PRACTICE

Tāḍāsana

Stand with your feet hip-width apart and parallel to each other. Rest your arms by your sides and allow your breath to be soft and wide. As you press into your heels, spread the skin and plantar fascia on the sole of your foot. Spread your toes like you are opening a paper fan. Keep your weight even on the four corners of both feet. Rock slightly forward onto the ball mounds of your big toes and little toes, then rock to the back edge of your heels. Continue swaying forward and back until you find the center between anterior and posterior shift. Then bend your knees thirty degrees and press your heels into the ground as you restraighten your legs. Charge and lift the inner seam of your legs from your inner ankles to your uppermost inner thighs. Lift your knees upward by engaging the front of your thighs. Hug the musculature of your leg close to the bone and sense your weight transmitting through the marrow of your bones.

Set a block between your upper thighs. As you squeeze the block, pull the side of your waist up away from the top of your pelvic rim. Avoid tightening or clenching your buttocks. Draw the flesh just below your navel back toward your spine and upward toward your head, like an updraft through a chimney flue. Float the back of your skull upward toward the ceiling and position the underside of your chin so that it is parallel to the floor. Sense an effortless balance in your skull and a feeling of equilibrium from ear to ear. Sense the polarity between the open crown at the top of your head and the open and wide surface at the soles of your feet. Avoid hardening anywhere in your pose; stand so your mountain is still, fluid, dynamic, and constantly changing. Stay for one to three minutes.

Take the block out and release out of the pose. Then practice tāḍāsana again, this time standing with your back against a wall. Bring your heels back to the base of the wall and touch the wall at your sacrum, shoulder blades, and back skull. The wall will give you feedback on your alignment, in particular how your pelvis, trunk, and skull stack over your feet. Hold for another minute.

The Mystical Midline

Now that we have discussed the foundation of the feet and the plumb line through the body, let us examine how the rest of the subtle and physical body is built on this foundation. The feet help orient to a sacred axis through the temple of the body, a pillar of self-organizing radiant vitality, revered in haṭha yoga as the primary pathway for the movement of the deepest life-force (kuṇḍalinī). Contemporary physiological renderings of this central axis involve the spine, spinal cord, and brain—that is, the central nervous system—yet we can imagine the central axis beginning in the inner foot. Like the subterranean veins of the earth that conduct the flow of mineral, water, and fire, the *nāḍīs* of the body travel from feet to spine and spine to feet. There are countless references to the central interior conduit, many of them marvelous analogies for the neurological plumb that conducts the flow of consciousness.

This central meridian has fascinating correlations to the formation of the spine during embryological development, for during the third week after conception, a primal midline appears within the matrix of burgeoning cells. This precursor to the spinal column emerges as a hollow shaft in the mesoderm, a middle germ layer of development that will house the neural tube. This midline is referred to in osteopathic medicine as the primitive streak, a central filament that evolves into the notochord and later the spinal cord. It is celebrated in mystical traditions as the placeholder for the body's deepest vitality.

One of the translations in yoga for this primal midline is *suṣumnā,* the "primary ray of the sun." This suggests that the animating pulse of life derives directly from solar energy. This luminous quality of the central channel is also known as *Chitriṇī*, the Lustrous or Radiant One. The central axis and all the nāḍīs in the body are aspects of an animating feminine power, and the word *Chitriṇī* implies erotic love, beauty, and rapture. Other epithets for the innermost channel are *Madhya Nāḍī* (the Middle Channel), *Śūnya Nāḍī* (the Empty Channel), *Nishabda Nāḍī* (the Silent Channel), and *Brahma Nāḍī* (the Channel of the godhead *Brāhma*). In any case, the axis mundi, the midline of the body, is charged with magnificence and power and is a source for both reverence and wonder.

The Lotus Feet

In the mystical yoga tradition, the chakras are likened to flowers that have the potential to bloom. Throughout this book we will investigate the metaphor of the root, stem, leaf, and flower of the lotus as it relates to the subtle body.

The stalk of a waterborne flower anchors itself in the earth and finds its nourishment in the muddy depths of ponds and lakes. The mud is the support and source of nourishment for the roots of the plant. In a similar way, the body finds its anchor and its stability at ground level, where the soles of the feet make contact with the earth.

There are numerous icons and statues from the yoga tradition that graphically depict the feet within an array of flower petals, demonstrating the notion that the entire body is supported on a lotus pad. Refer back to the tantric image featuring ritual implements on the sole of the foot—objects such as the *swastika*, a temple door, a half moon, Śiva in *padmāsana* (lotus pose), and the fortuitous six-pointed star (see fig. 1.4). In this mandala, the lotus feet are encoded with auspicious symbols that serve as guides to enlightenment through pathways within the subtle body.

In the natural world, the lotus stalk pumps nutrients from the sediment of the lake's fertile floor upward to its leaves and flower. Similarly, at the base of the body, the feet initiate a pumping, hydraulic movement up through the bones, connective tissues, and joints of the legs. For instance, when the feet are flexible and strong, they assist in good circulatory and metabolic activity throughout the ankles and knees. As the lotus feet *bloom* they encourage similar openings in the nervous system and subtle body, namely in and around the pelvis and sacrum. Because the feet tap the subterranean realm, they are the origin and source (called *mūla* in Sanskrit, meaning "root") for all becoming. In the yoga system they hold great potential and are considered sacred.

Feet of Honor

In India, a supreme act of devotion on the part of a spiritual aspirant is to touch the feet of the guru. This act of devotion is a gesture of reverence and respect. By touching (or kissing in demonstrative cases of extreme devotion) the feet of the teacher, the devotee is honoring the lineage of the teachings. Just as the feet transport the body in walking, the feet of the guru carry the tradition and the teachings down through generations. The feet are sacrosanct just as the *dharma,* the body of teachings, is sacred.

The opening verse of the Aṣṭāṅga Yoga Mantra begins, "Vande gurūnam charanaravinde," which translates into an homage to the lotus feet of all the ancestral teachers.[7]

In this invocation, the feet bear a kind of intelligence; they are full of power and sanctioned as placeholders of the tradition. Symbolically they transmit the teachings from one generation to the next. They are not everyday feet, but they hold potential for physio-spiritual awakening in the same way that the bud of the water lotus has the potential to bloom. The feet are charged with vitality (śakti), and their spiritual imprint on the path of yoga shows the way to liberation from suffering.

The soles of the feet and the crown of the head are uniquely paired. In one sense, the feet and crown are opposing as they are at extreme ends of the body. However, the feet and skullcap reciprocate as they form a dynamic balance between earth and sky. Within the subtle body, the feet and the head are storehouses for a treasury of wisdom. When a Hindu devotee touches the feet of the master and reciprocally touches his or her own forehead, it is a gesture that the wisdom of the lineage passes from teacher to student and from root to crown.

Washing of the Feet

When my younger brother, Michael, married Keerthi, a woman from South India, the wedding was held in Bangalore at the home of the bride's parents. During one of the initial stages of the wedding (weddings in India can be as long and complex as marriage itself), everyone in the wedding party had our feet washed by the bride's mother. This was a rare experience indeed for a Presbyterian family that hailed from a small New England town. I remember feeling both fascinated and slightly embarrassed at the prospect of having someone wash my feet in public, while decked out in fine wedding attire. Yet the ritual washing suggested a communal and familial cleansing, a kind of purification from the ground up. It was a way of paying tribute to and acknowledging the place or *stance* of the groom's family tree. Washing the feet was preparatory for the way the two families were to come together to stand on common ground. ◈

Sacred Seam of the Inside Leg

In yoga and classical ballet, the inside channels of the legs and arms designate connection to a divine current. By turning the feet and legs outward to an extreme, the inner lines of the leg—from toe point to pelvis—are expressed. Since its origins in fifteenth-century Europe and the age of the Renaissance, ballet has communicated, through movement and gesture, an affinity between God and humankind. Delicate and precise opening of the inner arms, legs, and ventral spine portray a rapport with a celestial, divine realm. Levity and grace are emphasized in positions such as the arabesque, relevé, and grand jeté. The interior pathways of the body in both classical ballet and haṭha yoga best articulate the flow of a noble and divine spirit.

This exaltation of the body's inner sleeves is consistent with anatomical connections within the leg and the body's core. The inner foot and inseam of the leg have myofascial continuity with the sanctum of the pelvic floor, iliopsoas, and ventral spine. Along the anterior spine, bundles of nerve plexuses congregate where the viscera are positioned. These are the chakras in yoga theory and practice, and extension of the inside leg incites movement within the chakras (discussed in the next chapter).

Stretching the connective tissues along the inner legs prompts flow within the nāḍīs. Anatomically, these are the femoral artery, vein, and nerve, lifelines to the leg that transit through the adductor muscles of the inner groin and wind down to the region of the inner heel.

Numerous poses stretch the inside leg—triangle pose, half moon pose, *vīrabhadrāsana II* or warrior pose II, and *baddha koṇāsana* or bound angle pose—and in so doing increase the flow of prāṇa into the legs (see fig. 2.3). The most classical of all yoga poses that harness the flow of the inside legs is *padmāsana*, the lotus pose, in which the inner legs are turned open like the petals of a flower and the ankles pressurize the inner groin region near the location of the femoral artery and nerve.

The Feet and Spinal Curves

In considering the body as an integrated whole, it is valuable to reflect on how the feet correlate to the spine. In the way that an infant is born without arches in her feet, there are no arches in the human spine at birth, only a posterior C-shape curve that the newborn retains from its embryonic journey. (Several yoga poses express this curve, including *piṇḍāsana* or embryo pose and bālāsana or child's pose.) This parabola-like arc of the spine is called a primary curve due to the fact that it is the first curve formed and it is shaped like a bow from head to tail. During embryological development, within the protected space of the spine's primary arc, the brain and internal organs mature and grow.

Cervical and lumbar curves—the secondary curves—develop in the spine by way of movement. The secondary curves are concave, meaning they bow into the body, and the alternating posterior-anterior curves give the spine its characteristic extensibility and spring. By way of the vertebral column's oppositional curves, it is able to gain its unique perpendicularity and at the same time bear the weight of the head and shoulder girdle. Biomechanically, the concave segments of the spine, the curves that develop through movement, are most prone to stress-related complications.

The first developmental curve to evolve is the cervical curve. In the first year, when the infant lays on his belly and begins to lift his hefty little head, the musculature at the base of the skull strengthens, thereby initiating arch within the cervical spine. In the process of pulling his head upward, he activates the musculature, ligaments, intervertebral disks, and spinal cord that pass through the cervical region.

This upward movement of the neck and skull initiates further neurovascular development within the brain and sensory organs. By leveraging his head off the crib floor, the infant begins its long journey upward against the force of gravity. This upward thrust of the head and neck against gravity resembles *bhujaṅgāsana* (cobra pose), one of the most classical of all haṭha yoga poses.

In yoga the upward rise of the cobra head suggests the upward push of consciousness. The impulse that prompts a baby to draw its head away from the ground is a remarkable example of the body's self-organizing instinct to evolve its awareness. Structurally the upthrust of the head involves not only the cervical spine but also the powerful musculature within the lower back. This extension of the lumbar spine is further developed in crawling. During the cross crawl, another critical connection—one between the arches of the feet and the lower back—occurs for postural development. The arch of the foot begins to develop spring, while the robust vertebrae of the lumbar spine move into the body. Note the parallel between the arches of the inner foot and the lumbar curve in the foot reflexology illustration (see fig 1.5). Similarly, in the pose *aṣṭāṅga namaskāra* (chest-knee-chin pose) below (see fig. 1.7), note the correlating curvature of the feet, low back, and neck.

Figure 1.7 Aṣṭāṅga Namaskāra and the Body's Anterior Curves

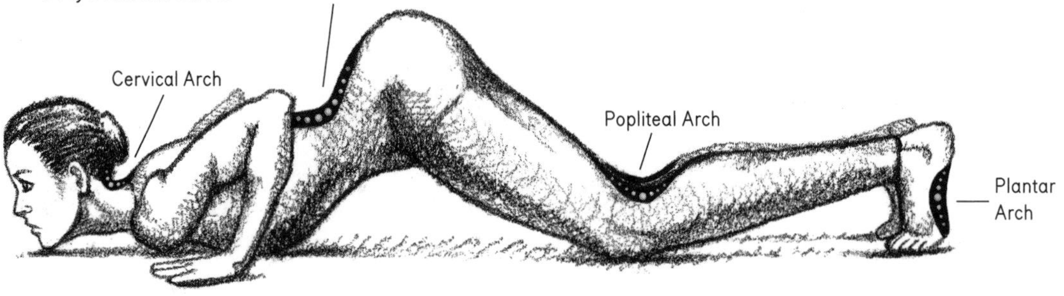

Connection between the foot arch, lumbar arch, and neck arch is important because, in keeping with the notion of building structural integrity from the ground up, we emphasize building the medial foot arch to secure the anterior spinal curves.

This structural reciprocity becomes crucial as we mature because many adults lose reinforcement in their arches. In yoga and other somatic disciplines, one of the primary aims is to generate greater structural integrity in the foot arches in order to help stabilize the lower back. If the arches of the feet collapse or fall, then the lower back may compress. Lower back pain is endemic in our culture—85 percent of the population experiences back pain.[8]

Laxity within the soft tissues (ligaments, tendons, and musculature) of the ankles and feet, combined with lack of exercise and excess weight, may contribute to prolapse of the internal organs. If the organs such as the uterus, bladder, or colon do not receive sufficient support from the feet, legs, and surrounding pelvic musculature, they can droop toward the pelvic floor. If the gut drapes toward the pelvic floor, a multitude of potential ailments may arise, as we will see in the next chapter. Developing spring and resilience in the soles of the feet helps to provide the structural integrity for the internal organs within the pelvic cavity and in the region of the low back.

PRACTICE

Sūryanamaskāra and the Chest-Knee-Chin Pose

This pose is called *aṣṭāṅga namaskāra,* the chest-knee-chin pose, typically done as part of a *sūryanamaskāra,* or a sun salutation sequence. It suggests prostration as it is done prone with eight points (*aṣṭāṅga*) touching the floor—the two feet, knees, and hands plus the sternum and chin. It is an older version of the more athletic *chaturaṅga daṇḍāsana* (four-limbed staff pose) and much more accessible. This pose helps develop concavity in the arch of the foot, the arch within the lumbar spine, and the arch within the neck.

Begin in tāḍāsana and with an inhale, launch your arms upward. With the exhale, fold down toward your feet. Breathe in again as you raise your head and trunk upward and exhale to step back into a high push-up position with your arms straight and your

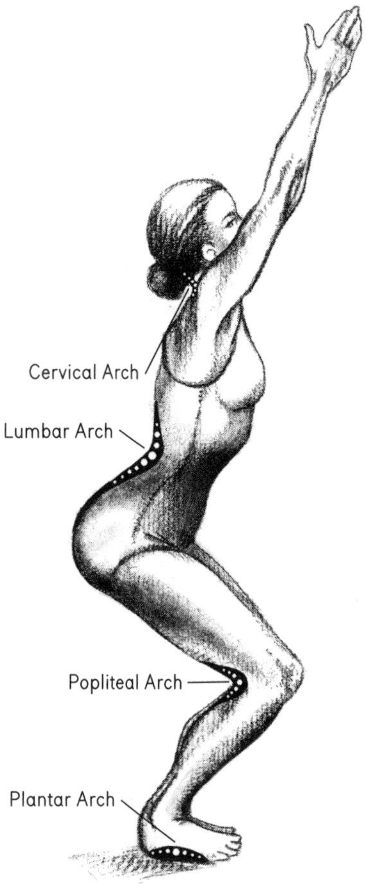

Figure 1.8 Utkaṭāsana, Spinal Curves, and the Arch of the Foot

toes turned under as in the broken-toe pose variation of vajrāsana. Then lower your knees, sternum, and chin to the floor. Keep your toes in flexion and press your toes into the floor to activate the arches in your feet. At the same time, spike your buttock bones upward into the air to actively create a lumbar curve in your lower back. In particular, sense the way your fifth lumbar vertebra (L5) moves forward into your body, away from your sacrum (see fig. 3.3, model B). Remain for thirty seconds to a minute breathing normally.

Balance on the midpoint of your sternum and chin. Observe the movement of your cervical curve in tandem with your lumbar arch and plantar "arch." Retract your shoulders away from your ears and press firmly into the base of your thumb and forefinger. Within your pose, sense and feel the correlation of the convex shapes in your feet, back of knees, lumbar, and neck. Gaze softly down the tip of your nose and in toward the midline of your body.

From the aṣṭāṅga namaskāra position, slither forward into the cobra, then push back to downward-facing dog pose. After thirty seconds to a minute, step or jump your feet to your hands. Inhale and reach up with straight legs, then exhale and fold down. Then with your feet together, bend your knees and enter *utkaṭāsana* (fierce pose). This pose rigorously combines activation of the foot, lumbar, and cervical curves. Allow your trunk to lean forward thirty degrees from the midline. Activate the arches of your feet by pressing into the four corners on the sole of each foot. Simultaneously create a concavity in your lumbar spine and look slightly upward in order to generate a gentle concavity in your neck (fig. 1.8). Then with the exhalation, push into your feet, rise upward, and return to tāḍāsana.

Pada Bandha

There is a dynamic polarity between the diaphragm at the sole of the foot and the perineum at the base of the spine. The reciprocity of the two diaphragms stems from the architectural symmetry between the root support at the base of the leg and the support at the base of the spine. Both uphold bony scaffolding—the feet support the tibia, fibula, and femur and the perineum supports the spine and pelvis.

There is coordination of these two diaphragms. Mūla bandha, the root bind, traditionally thought to be isolated in the pelvic floor, commences with the lifting of the muscular padding at the sole of the foot. In haṭha yoga, mūla bandha is considered to be the pivotal movement that draws the kuṇḍalinī upward through the spine. Engagement at the sole of the foot is sometimes referred to as *pada bandha;* it supports mula bandha in establishing a flow of kinetic forces upward through the body.

Pada means "foot," and *bandha* means a bind, hold, catch, latch, fasten, or tether. In yoga practice bandha suggests an interior harness or yoke, to animate the flow of prāṇa. Lifting the first diaphragm within the foot via pada bandha provides core lift through the bony matrix of the leg.[9] Pada bandha includes lift of the medial, lateral, and transverse arches and leverage of the center of the sole of the foot. Activation of this focal point at midfoot stimulates a vital *marma* point (marma points in Ayurveda are like acupressure points in traditional Chinese medicine) called the *tala hṛdaya* (see fig. 1.2). *Tala* means "surface," and *hṛdaya* means "heart." Thus, pada bandha involves lift of the "heart of the foot."

PRACTICE

Pressure Point Release on the Sole of the Foot

In order to stimulate the pressure points on the sole of the foot, including tala hṛdaya, sit in *virāsana* (pose of virility). Make a fist with your hands and press your knuckles into the soles of your feet. Begin near the heel in the region where your plantar fascia attaches to your anterior heel. In foot reflexology, this area corresponds to the large intestine. When there is intestinal disorder, the referral points near the heel are sensitive and painful. Notice the colon (large intestine) adjacent to the heel in the foot reflexology drawing in figure 1.5.

Slide your knuckles to the midfoot. If you land on the very center of your foot, you are pressing on the tala hṛdaya (also called *pada madhya*, the Middle of the Foot point). This point is used to provide grounding when experiencing stress, agitation, or anxiety. This center of the sole of the foot corresponds to the kidney and respiratory diaphragm. Press your knuckles into the thick padding of your center foot in order to stimulate the flow of prāṇa in your kidneys.

Direct pressure can be accomplished by standing on a tennis ball or, for more exacting pressure, a golf ball. This can be done instead of the knuckle pressure onto the sole of the foot in virāsana. Stand on one leg while placing the ball under the sole of your other foot. Rest your hand against the wall or table in order to secure your balance. When stepping onto the ball, it is good to *pump* the tissues on the sole of your foot by first sinking into the ball and then releasing the pressure. Reposition the ball periodically so that the pressure is distributed across the sole of your foot.

Then stand in tāḍāsana and press down the four corners of your foot. As you do so, draw the center of the sole of your foot upward, as if elevated by a string. Imagine you are a marionette and that the string inserts into the tala hṛdaya. Visualize the pull of the marionette string providing leverage for your midfoot. Observe whether your posture feels more buoyant and lifted following the pressure point stimulation on the soles of your feet.

The Wellspring of the Foot

Near the center of the foot and slightly toward the toes from the tala hṛdaya point is a critical acupressure point in traditional Chinese medicine (TCM) that initiates flow within the body. Called Kidney 1, this point in Chinese medicine theory is delightfully named the Gushing Spring, or Wellspring, for it is thought to nourish the kidney chi. It is the lowest acupressure point in the entire body. Anatomically, the kidneys are located just below the respiratory diaphragm in the upper solar plexus.

In TCM and qigong, the kidneys are the reservoirs for life's vitality and govern our most inherent levels of activity (yang) and rest (yin). We will see in chapter 4 the importance of the kidneys to the subtle body. In the same way that a spring along a mountain slope or in a meadow provides nourishment, Kidney 1 is a source point for the flow of the essential life-force. According to Peter Deadman and Mazin Al-Khafaji, "Kidney 1 point is an important point in qigong practice. Directing the mind to Kidney 1, or inhaling and exhaling through this point, roots and descends the chi in the lower *dan tian* (cinnabar field) and helps the body absorb the yin energy of the earth."[10] (See fig. 1.5.) Pressure on this point in TCM is used to reduce swelling in the foot, counter neuropathy, and lessen chronic pain and numbness. In both yoga and qigong, standing poses enable the practitioner to cultivate the flow of chi or prāṇa from the base. The Taoist sage Chuang Tzu once said "the true man breathes from his feet up, while ordinary people just breathe from the throat."[11] This suggests that the font of life, the wellspring of prāṇa, begins in the foot.

Thresholds to the Subtle Body

In yoga the soles of the feet and the palms of the hands function like chakras, awakening prāṇa currents that flow through the arms, legs, and spine. We can imagine the feet to be the first chakra, as they prompt movement from the ground upward through the body. When we activate the feet, we begin to activate the bioenergy of the chakra system.

The soles of the feet and the palms of the hands together are thresholds to the subtle body. In the way that bandhas release energy along the spine, peripheral points of the hands and feet mobilize flow through the nāḍīs of the extremities. Considered portals to awakening, the palms and soles of the feet ready the mind for meditation and states of yogic concentration (*samādhi*).

One Tibetan *tangka* (a sacred scroll) of an enlightened lama demonstrates this concept. It features a robed figure in a celestial tree canopy in the center of the scroll, and flanking him are drawings of human hands and feet. They are large in scale and gold-hued, and in the center of each hand and foot is a sketch of the wheel of the dharma. The *dharma chakra* is well known for having been first set in motion by Shākyamuni Buddha to help guide students in the process of awakening to the unconfined nature of mind. Thus, the dharma wheels in the palmar and plantar centers are openings to meditative states of awareness.

Rivers of the Subtle Body

In many respects, a yoga practice should begin by opening the hands and feet while strengthening the peripheral joints of the ankles and wrists. It is through the soles of our feet and palms of our hands that we interface with the world. By opening the distal points of the body—in particular spreading the hands and fingers as well as the feet and toes—we create a corresponding connection to the proximal points within the core of the body. That is, we access the core from the periphery. When opening the distal points of the hands and feet, we also gain a better sense of our personal boundaries and limits.

In the acupuncture theory of traditional Chinese medicine, meridians begin or terminate their flow at distal points in the hands and feet. Like in yoga, where prāṇa is thought to flow through tubular channels called nāḍīs (rivers), in TCM, the chi or *jing* transits through meridians. Jing is the essential substance that courses through the body and enlivens all tissues. Jing is thought to flow along interior rivers (called *jingluo*). In the subtle body, the principal "river" in the body is the spine along with its spinal cord. Knowing that the body's essential vitality moves via fluid dynamics, practitioners of the internal arts relied on farming analogies to articulate the flow of internal prāṇa or chi. Thus, nāḍīs and meridians are likened to internal waterways. The body's vital force, while invisible to the eye, is palpable to those who collect and channel its movement.

At the distal tips of the fingers and toes, the chi surfaces and flows. It moves proximally through shallow, delicate tributaries. In meridian theory of TCM, chi begins to percolate from the periphery at what are called the jing-well points. In the way water emerges from an aquifer, the chi surfaces at the body's periphery and trickles through meridian rivulets. These tributaries trickle at the toes and fingertips, flow through the ankles and wrists, and proceed via points at the knees and elbows to plunge deeper into the body (fig. 1.9). In reference to the flow of chi in the extremities (referred to as "qi" in the excerpt below), the *Spiritual Pivot,* a textbook of TCM compiled around the first century B.C.E., states:

> The point at which the qi rises is known as the jing-well. The point at which the qi glides is known as the ying-spring. The point at which the qi pours though is known as the shu-stream. The point at which the qi flows is known as the jing-river. The point at which the qi enters inwards is known as the he-sea.[12]

The image of moving water signifying the vital life-force is evident. Where the meridians pass through the elbow or knee (the *he-sea* points, or "uniting points") en route to the organs deeper inside the torso, the meridians plummet deep into the body. Figure 1.9 shows the spleen meridian passing from foot to inside knee. By actively stretching this channel in a pose such as pārśvakonāsana, the internal organs are stimulated. It is important to remember that by stimulating the peripheral points at the toe tips, fingertips,

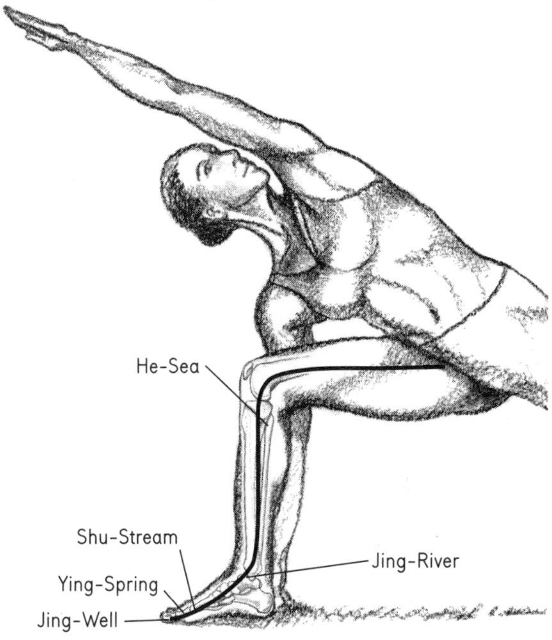
He-Sea
Shu-Stream
Jing-River
Ying-Spring
Jing-Well

Figure 1.9 Points in the Meridian Stream (Spleen Channel)

ankles, and wrists you can impart an energetic current of chi to the body's core. Once the distal feet and legs are open, a river of unobstructed flow can pass into the pelvis and sacrum. The flow of these vapory, exquisitely fine streams nourishes the organs, glands, and spinal nerves. We now turn to the structures within the pelvis that provide support for the long, deep river of the spine.

PRACTICE

Opening the Eyes of the Toes

This practice serves to build elasticity and increase proprioceptive awareness in the toes. This will improve balance and provide an overall sense of stability in standing and walking.

While standing in tāḍāsana, set your feet hip-width apart. Raise your toes off the floor and extend all ten forward, like baby turtles pulling their heads out of their shells to look around. At the same time plant the front two corners of your feet at the base of the little toe and base of the big toe. As you set your toes down see if you can individuate the length of each toe, starting with the baby toe, then the ring toe, the middle toe, the index toe, and the big toe. Create a space between each toe as if you have webbing between your toes.

Actively reach the necks of your toes forward toward the front of your mat, thereby activating the tributaries of chi flow. Lift your toes once again away from the floor and as you set them down imagine you are resting them on a piece of tracing paper, touching lightly so that you will not indent the paper. Feel a spherical opening at the very tip of your toes and imagine you have ten eyes, one at the end of each toe. Open these toe eyes wide and clear. Recall that the toes and toe tips refer to the eyes in foot reflexology (see fig. 1.5). At the same time (with your cranial eyes) gaze softly to a point on the horizon. Relax the membrane covering your eyeballs and soften the skin at the inner and outer edges of your eye. As you gaze toward a single point in front of you (and slightly down), observe everything within a 180-degree arc. Your peripheral gaze will help keep your brain quiet but focused. Maintain a soft, steady awareness in both your toe eyes and cranial eyes. Remain for two minutes. Afterward, transition into downward dog and follow with a series of standing poses with a similar focus.

2

THE PELVIS POTENTIAL

Unlocking the Power of the Spine

We shall not cease from exploration
And the end of all of our exploring
Will be to arrive where we started
And to know the place for the first time.
Through the unknown, remembered gate . . .
At the source of the longest river . . .
—T. S. Eliot, "Little Gidding"[1]

The spinal base is the "source of the longest river," a river of tremendous strength and potential that flows through the spinal shaft. Its flow is harnessed by movements within the pelvic floor and subtle articulations of the coccyx. We begin to navigate the course of this spinal river from the tailbone and perineum. Like the keel of a boat, the pelvis provides stability to the spine and counterweight to the cranium. For this reason, it is important to align and balance the pelvis, not an easy task given the kinds of compressive forces typically loaded onto the spinal base. Yet movement in the hip sockets, tailbone, and pelvic floor allow for muscular and neuro-vascular flow between the legs, trunk, and cranium. It is by unblocking the rigidity and congestion in the first chakra, the mūlādhāra chakra, that the sublime channels within the subtle body can flow without obstruction.

The Artistry of the Pelvis

The spherical design of the pelvis is beautiful. Its soaring arches, curvaceous borders, and hidden notches have inspired artists like Georgia O'Keeffe to paint its magnificent contours. The architecture of the pelvis, with its vaulted circular crests, is at once earthy and celestial. Like canyon walls, the ridges of the pelvis shelter and define the rivers that meander through it. The ilia resemble wings that spread as they climb. Their protective sphere provides a sanctuary for the body's central channels.

Anatomically, the outward flare of the two semicircular hemispheres of the pelvis provide span and depth in order to house the pelvic organs along with the vessels and nerves that transit from the abdomen to the legs. As the wings of the pelvis arch upward, they twist, and the artistry of this form adds to its sculptural beauty. The whorl within the pelvic bones contributes to the spiral-like motion of the deep life-force that pumps throughout the entire body.

The curved edges of the upper ilia have multiple attachment sites for muscles that sweep down from the abdomen and for muscles that climb upward from the sides of the legs. Like a railroad switchyard, where train tracks converge onto a multidirectional hub that pivots, the curve of each ilium enables a broad range of motion in the leg, hip socket, and side waist. Contributing to this range of motion, muscle fibers on the outside pelvis, such as the gluteus medius muscle, twirl and flare. The three-dimensional curl of the ilia is impossible to appreciate when drawn on paper and best to experience in movement. The spiralic shapes in and around the pelvis contribute to the serpentine flow of the kuṇḍalinī force.

The soaring arches of the ilia form a chute that funnels down to the pelvic basin at the tip of the tail bone. Where the pelvis tapers at its base, it forms a partial sphere that in many ways mirrors the shape of the cranium. So it is possible to imagine that we have two skulls: the cranium at the top of the spine, which is a nearly completely closed orb, and the pelvis at the base, which is enclosed on its sides but open at its superior and inferior ends. The two spheres are synchronistic in their movements. In this chapter we will see how the sacrum that forms the back of the pelvis and the occiput that comprises the posterior cranium articulate as part of the craniosacral system. We typically think that aptitude is invested in the cranium alone, but the pelvic *skull* also houses a kind of intelligence. In yoga, this intelligence is far below the machinations of the rational brain, concentrated in the instinctual power of the kuṇḍalinī.

Drinking from the Wine Cup

Evolutionarily, standing upright on two legs is a remarkable phenomenon. Bipedalism is something we take for granted, yet standing presents real challenges. Structurally, locomotion is easier and more efficient on four legs rather than two, due to the way that forces are distributed between pelvic and shoulder girdles in the four-legged posture. Thus, it is easier for coyotes, reindeer, and pumas to maintain a balanced spine.

Standing on two legs is akin to standing on stilts, for our center of gravity is propped upward, far from the ground. As a result, kinetic forces typically become bottled up in the hip joint. In yoga, hip openers that involve external rotation serve to stretch and strengthen the fan-shaped muscles that radiate out along the outer hip. The task of loosening constriction in the hip region is, for most students, the most painstaking (and painful!) part of the yoga practice.

The design of the uppermost femur is unique to bipeds, for the thighbone achieves virtually a right angle at its proximal end, where it angles into the hip socket. This is called the neck of the femur, and like the cervical spine, this upper femur can be a real pain in the neck.

Fortunately, the hip socket, a spherical enclosure that houses the ball of the femur, is entirely cushioned by cartilage. This cartilage is like the rubberized, spongy surface of an indoor tennis court or track and field facility—rigid but with some give. The ball bearing of the femur head is further cushioned and lubricated by a viscous liquid called synovial fluid.

The ligaments that span the hip joint (iliofemoral ligaments) by necessity are strapping and robust: they are some of the strongest ligaments in the body (fig. 2.1). Like the vaulting arches of the ilia, these ligaments spiral as they form a snug wreath around the ball and socket joint. The iliofemoral ligaments have the resilience of a wet and twisted towel—a structure that has give yet is extremely difficult to tear. Their strength and resilience are necessary to secure the femur head into the

Figure 2.1 Sacrum and Piriformis

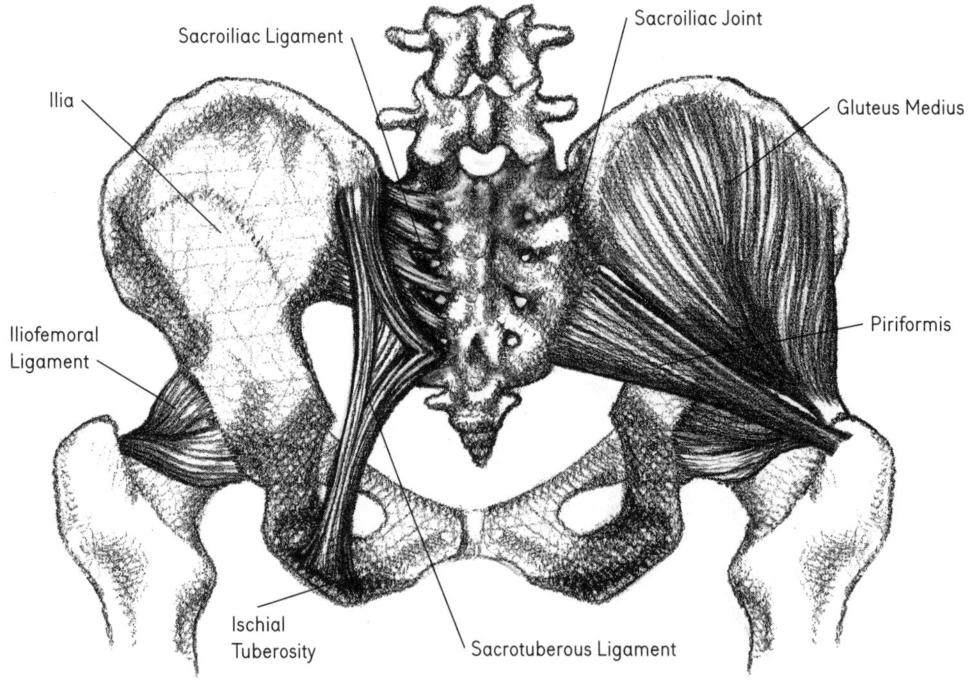

cup-shaped hip joint. Rigidity of the iliofemoral ligaments is in part what restricts students in deep hip openers. For people who have been athletic—runners, soccer players, and hikers—accumulated compression frequently amasses in their hip joint muscle and ligaments.

The fossa of the hip socket that receives the ball of the femur is shaped like a chalice. Called the acetabulum, the concave surface of the hip joint was so named because it resembled a wine or vinegar cup used in Greek and Roman times. The wine-cup analogy is a possible reference to the subtle body. If the structures around the hip joint are mobile, a flow of essential fluids—blood, lymph, and cerebrospinal fluid—can pass unimpeded through the pelvis, and in turn affect buoyancy deep within the spine. We can imagine the flow of an inebriating libation through the body to be like the flow of ambrosia or nectar. In Indian lore, as in Greek mythology, a semidivine fluid was thought to flow like an eternal spring through the body and was thought to be a source of both longevity and immortality. In the pelvis, when the ball of the femur in the hip joint swivels and turns, it helps propel the life-sustaining inner fluids. In the way that winemakers press grapes in order to make wine, poses such as padmāsana (lotus pose), *gomukhāsana* (cow pose), and *kandāsana* (pose of the bulbous root) are positions that serve to *press the nectar* in and around the hips and prompt effervescent pulsations within the spine (fig. 2.2).

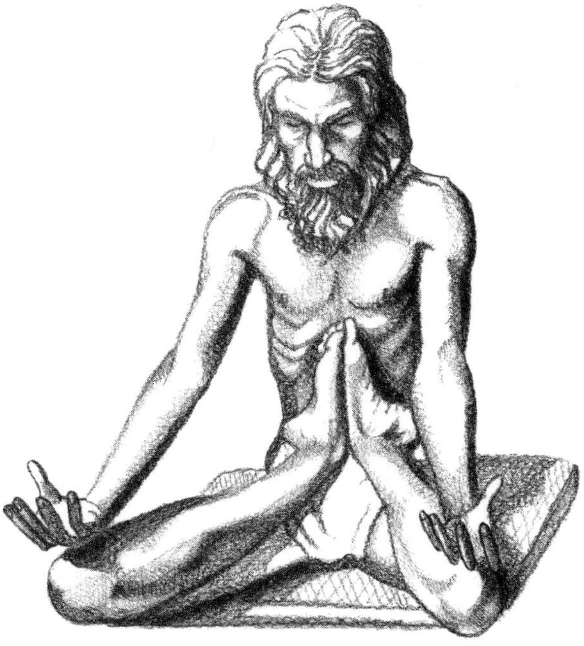

Figure 2.2 Yogi in Kandāsana

The Spherical Head of the Femur

The hip joint is often a zone of significant compression and tension. The super-snug fit of the femoral head, vacuum packed into the suction cup of the hip socket (the acetabular labrum), often becomes distressed on one or both sides. The entire complex of the hip and buttock muscles is frequently tighter on one side causing asymmetry. The hip sockets may assume different characteristics, or *personalities*, right to left, due to trauma, genetics, repetitive strain, short-legged syndrome, or postural traits whereby one leg assumes the burden of weight more than the other. In light of chronic asymmetrical holding, one hip may slip, shear, or catch. When the hip joints are uneven, it is comparable to an automobile with poor alignment and can cause the entire physical structure to veer or pull to one side. Repeated pulling to one side can aggravate the ligaments and labrum in one or both hip sockets. If chronic displacement causes painful restriction in the encapsulating rings of ligament around the hip socket, then the individual may be a candidate for hip replacement.

Stabilizing the Hip

I encourage students to discern which of their hip joints has more or less give. Sometimes imbalance is due to gluing in the myofascia around the hip, and sometimes it is due to excess laxity. A joint with too much play or mobility can be as problematic as a restricted one, especially in the hip, given the load-bearing demand on the hip sockets.

To stabilize and secure the ball and socket complex of the hip, we need to anchor the head of the femur firmly in the hip socket. Like the way a vice fastens a structure between its jaws, the spherical head of the femur is pinned to the hip joint. Standing poses like trikoṇāsana (triangle pose), pārśvakoṇāsana (flank pose), and *vīrabhadrāsana* I and II (warrior pose I and II) help to generate bilateral symmetry in the hip sockets. One-legged balancing poses such as vṛkṣāsana (tree pose) and ardha chandrāsana (half moon pose) are especially helpful in aligning and building sturdiness in the weight-bearing hip joint

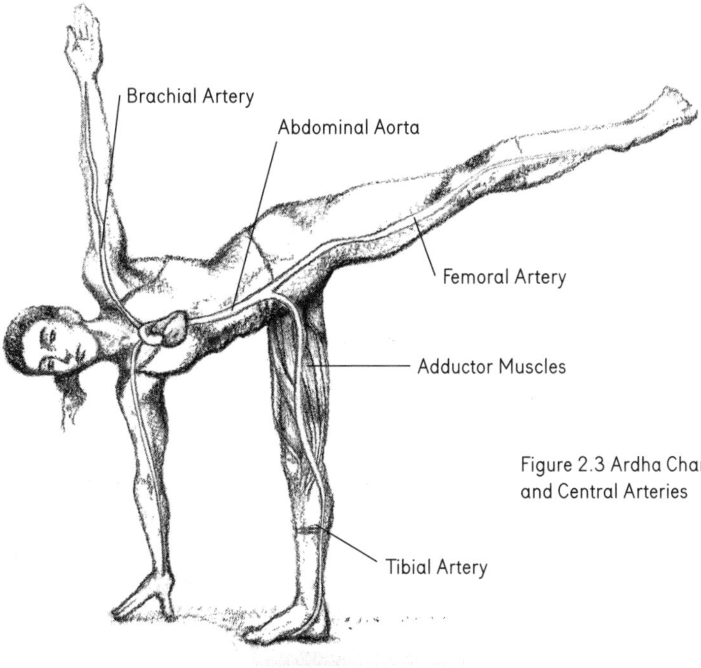

Figure 2.3 Ardha Chandrāsana and Central Arteries

(see fig. 2.3). This securing of the femoral heads generates stability for the entire pelvis and spine. The vice grip action of the hip sockets aids in cases of osteoporosis, as the ligaments and tendons around the hip joints are strengthened and the bony matrix within the femur and pelvic bones is deliberately stressed. Bearing weight through the bones aids in building greater bone density and increases absorption of calcium into the bones.

Physiologically, the marrow of the long bones of the femurs and the marrow of the ilia (hip bones) are critical production sites for red blood cells in the body (especially in the growing years). In both Āyurveda and Chinese medicine, bone marrow is equated with the body's quintessential life spirit. Thus, the significance of the thighbone is not limited to its physical properties. Over the course of history in certain tantric rituals of India and Tibet, the ancestral femur bone is prized as a relic and is charged with spiritual power.

The Christmas Tree Stand

I think of the stability generated in the hip sockets through standing poses as the Christmas tree stand. If you have ever attempted to set up a cut Christmas tree in a stand equipped with metal screws, you know the challenge of erecting the tree on the vertical. The task of getting the Christmas tree to stay upright so that it doesn't tip over onto the dining room table, sending glasses of eggnog flying, is like the challenge of standing efficiently in samasthiti (even standing pose). Securing the outer femurs evenly into the hip sockets in order to support the erect spine is akin to fastening the metal screws to the circumference of the tree base. Tightening the screws toward the midline enables the tree to balance vertically. Fortunately, the tree stand has at least three screws, yet people have only two hip sockets. This suggests how difficult it is to truly stand efficiently. However, unlike the stationary Christmas tree, the ball and socket joint of the human hip is mobile and designed to accommodate strain by distributing forces into the surrounding soft tissues.

Improving stability in the pelvis is gained by increasing elasticity and strength in musculature that forms the hip socket, primarily the piriformis muscle and the gluteus medius. However, this should not involve clenching or gripping the buttock muscles. While the head of the femur is secure in the hip joint, the gluteal muscles should remain pliable and adaptable. The buttock muscles are prone to hypertonicity, so most hip openers in yoga aim to lengthen and broaden the abductor muscles that serve to externally rotate the leg. The piriformis muscle is a key component of the hip complex. It is an *inside-out* muscle, for its broad end attaches intrinsically to the anterior sacrum, while its narrower end attaches laterally to the greater trochanter (fig. 2.1). The word *piriformis* stems from the Latin *pirum,* meaning "pear," and *forma,* meaning "shape." Thus, the muscle is wide, like the belly of a pear, where it attaches to the sacrum and becomes narrow where it adheres to the trochanter. It forms the upper margin of the pelvic floor complex where it attaches to the sacrum. When the piriformis muscle is constricted, it may yank the sacrum out of center and thus contribute to sacroiliac dysfunction.

The piriformis muscle is usually complicit when there is sciatic pain, for the sciatic nerve transits directly underneath the piriformis muscle. Nerve entrapment of the sciatic nerve is linked to piriformis syndrome, which can cause pain in "the low back, groin, perineum, buttock, hip, posterior thigh and leg, foot, and, during defecation, in the rectum."[2]

For modern-day practitioners it can be a lifelong project to achieve fluidity and balance through the hip joints. When the hip capsules are both supple and stable and you can revolve your hips in profound hip-opening āsana, the nāḍīs are pressed and a divine nectar, referred to as *amṛta,* is thought to flow. In this way you are thought to have longevity paralleled only by the gods.

PRACTICE

Hip Awareness: Three Exercises

The following three exercises help bring awareness to the structures in and around the hip socket: The first serves to increase range of motion without weight bearing. The second actively stretches the lateral hip muscles. And the last, tree pose, brings stability to the hip via load bearing. In each of the movements, begin to discern which of your hip sockets is more restricted. In this way you will gain greater somatic intelligence and will become more attuned to the subtle pulls, torques, and shifts within your structure. By noticing how your hips differ, you can distinguish which side needs to be strengthened and which side needs to be released. Be curious about getting to know your own body. Have the intention to achieve greater symmetry.

Circular Flow in the Hip Sockets

This series of movements brings fluidity and ease of motion to the hip sockets. It also helps assess imbalances and asymmetrical patterns in the ligaments and musculature of the hip joint and sacral area. Practice the movements slowly and initiate the movement from the rotation of your hip socket, less from the musculature of your leg. Sense and feel the circular fluidity of your hip joint capsules.

Lie onto your back and relax as in śavāsana. Externally rotate the femur in your hip socket and draw one leg up into the tree pose shape. Keep your foot on the floor and glide your knee out to the side and close to the floor. Then slide the leg back out to śavāsana, initiating the movement from the swivel-like action of your hip socket. Repeat five to eight times on one side. Then repeat the same movement on the other side, so that the *slide and glide* is done slowly and without force. Do not hold the position, but glide in and out, taking your leg along the floor to tree pose and then sliding it back out straight. As you proceed, compare the two sides: Is one side more sticky or loose? Do you feel a catch on one side? Is the limitation of movement on the inside of your hip socket or the outside?

The next phase of the exercise takes the hip socket into a half-circle movement. Again slide your bent knee out to the side on the floor into external rotation. Then plant the foot of that leg into the floor and gently draw your knee up toward the ceiling. Then arc your knee across the midline of your body, so that your knee and hip move into internal rotation. At this point your outer hip will lift several inches from the floor. Then from the internal angle of your knee and hip, slide your foot back out to śavāsana. Keep your foot in contact with the floor the entire time. Repeat on the other side. This movement describes a circular rotation of your hip joint combining external rotation, flexion, internal rotation, and extension of your hip. Alternate this movement on both your right and left sides. Do five to seven sets. Again compare your two sides. Should you detect an imbalance, it can inform you as to how to organize your yoga practice. When there is laxity in the hip socket aim to strengthen and secure your hip. When there is constriction, practice to create greater mobility. As you make these circular movements, visualize synovial fluid lubricating your hip joint. This will help hydrate and bring nutrition into the joint capsule.

Drawing Nectar from the Pear

To stretch the piriformis and draw juice (amṛta) from the pear-shaped muscle at the back of your pelvis, place your legs into *sukhāsana* (contentment pose). Be sure that your feet are set directly underneath your knees, not against your thighs. Position your legs so that your shins are approximately parallel to the front edge of your mat. Bend forward by lengthening your side waist and elongating the front edge of your spine. As you fold, rest your forehead on the floor, a block, or bolster. Lightly flex your feet. Feel your buttock muscles spread and feel the stretch of your piriformis. Hold for two to three minutes. To come up, bring your hands to the floor near your knees and push to rise upward. Repeat by reversing your legs so your other shin is in front. Compare each side of your body for the amount of tension held in your piriformis muscle and hip joint. Recollect the laxity or tension you detected in the "Circular Flow in the Hip Sockets" exercise. Notice the ways in which you encounter the same constellation of holding in your hip joint and surrounding musculature.

Standing Tree

Stand in vṛkṣāsana (tree pose) and bring awareness to your standing leg. Sink your standing heel into the floor and actively lift the inner arch of your standing foot. Raise your opposite foot and plant it securely and as high as possible along the inside edge of your standing leg. Press the foot of your bent leg firmly into the inner bank of your standing leg thigh. This will help increase blood flow through your femoral artery and groin muscles. At the same time extend the inside of your raised leg away from your midline. Notice how the hip socket of your standing leg tends to displace to the side, and your entire pelvis shifts away from the bent knee. Secure and stabilize your pose by drawing the head of the femur into the socket on your standing leg side, like the Christmas tree technique. Attempt to align and center the hip joint of your standing leg directly over your ankle. Feel how securing the head of the femur solidifies your tree pose and works like a mini bandha. Avoid clenching your buttocks or tightening your pelvic floor. Secure the posture with the vice-like pressure of the greater trochanters on the outside of your hips. Hold each side for one to two minutes.

Sacred Inner Channels: Nāḍīs of the Leg

The inside leg and pelvis are much different from the exterior hip and leg, for along the inside bank of the pelvis passes a large neurovascular bundle. Inner rivers of blood, lymph, and nerve emerge from deep within the abdomen, course alongside the navel, and dive downward through the interior pelvis. The iliac nerve, artery, and vein are carefully cached and protected by the walls of the ilia; they are lifelines, transporting nerve signals and blood to the leg. Exiting the pelvis, they transit through the upper groins, and tunnel down the inside channel of the leg as the femoral arteries, veins, and nerves (fig. 2.3). If the iliac and femoral arteries were positioned on the lateral hip or leg, they would be vulnerable to rupture—should one of these blood lines be severed, you would bleed to death within minutes.

Along with blood and nerve flow, the inside hip and thigh harbor a colony of lymph nodes called the inguinal lymph nodes. Lymph that drains from the foot and lower leg follows a course along the inside channel of the femur. Lymph flows through the upper inner thigh, along the interior pelvis, and into the abdominal region.

As we saw in the last chapter, these circulatory and neurological channels are part of the body's sacred interior. Yoga postures such as half moon pose serve to open these conduits, effectively modifying blood pressure, heart rate, the circulation of lymph, respiratory rhythms, and consciousness. After stretching and opening the *extrinsic* musculature along the outer leg and hip, the yogi aims to stretch and strengthen the *intrinsic* musculature along the inner leg and hip. This involves building length and strength in the adductor muscles of the legs (the inner groins) and the all-important iliopsoas muscle. In the Iyengar system of yoga there are innumerable cues given to access and activate the inner groins—the back groins, the top groins, the upper and inner groins, and so on. To open the myofascial compartment of the inner thigh is to open the core sheath of the body. This serves to improve the flow of blood and nerve impulses that travel between the hip and leg.

Poses that passively restore the inner leg such as *supta baddha koṇāsana* (reclined bound angle pose), *supta pādāṅguṣṭāsana* (reclining big toe pose), and a variation of *viparīta karanī* (legs-up-the-wall pose) with legs set in baddha koṇāsana, are therapeutic as they open the nāḍīs that transit down the inner thigh. They increase the circulation of blood and lymph and improve neurological flow through the pelvis, down the leg, and into the foot. Passive opening of the inner leg also acts as a tonic for the yin meridians in traditional Chinese medicine that course along the inner thigh, namely the liver, kidney, and spleen channels (see fig. 4.2). Thus, supported poses that drape open the inner legs have a profound restorative effect on the subtle body. I often say to my students who are studying therapeutic yoga, if the inside leg and pelvis are supported and lengthened, it will undoubtedly facilitate the healing process. This is particularly important since the inner legs and pelvis are often blocked and congested due to postural restrictions and emotional holding.

The Heels of the Pelvis

As we continue to travel the body from the ground upward, we now turn our attention to the bony structures at the very base of the pelvis. The dynamic and curved wings of the ilia attach to the underlying pelvic bones called the ischia. These dense and compact bones are the lowest struts within the architecture of the pelvis. The sitting bones are knobby protrusions, and their thick and bony mass adds weight and stability to the pelvis, like ballast in the hull of a boat. They are important guides for determining how to bear weight in seated poses. The sitting bones, called the ischial tuberosities (one of my favorite anatomical terms), are most likely the structures that are supporting you right now as you read (see fig. 2.1).

It is easy to imagine that the sitting bones are cousins to the heels in terms of form and function. Just as the heel of the foot supports the weight of the leg, the *heel* of the sitting bone supports the weight of the spine and pelvis. Both are spherical, heavy, and rigid. They both make contact with a supporting surface—the heels to the floor in standing, the sitting bones to the cushion or mat when seated—and so are crucial points of reference for assessing how weight gets distributed side to side. (We will explore a third set of *heels* at the base of the skull, the occipital condyles, in chapter 7.)

In postural training, it is important to observe how the sitting bones make contact with the floor. If one side of the pelvis bears more weight when sitting, then the entire pelvis and spine may pitch to the side. Check your posture now to see whether you are leaning more onto one sitting bone and research whether you chronically tip onto one buttock bone when sitting. It is common when sitting at work or eating dinner for the weight of the body to routinely teeter to one side. Chronic displacement to one side can cause compression in the hip, foreshorten the lower back, and possibly contribute to scoliotic curvature of the spine.

In the last chapter, in light of Śiva's trident and the three prongs of the heel, we examined how weight falls into the heel when standing (see fig 1.3). When seated, it is helpful to do a similar assessment: Where is the weight on my sitting bones? Am I resting on the back edge or front edge of the buttock bones? Am I on the inner or outer edge of my sitting bone? How weight is borne by the sitting bones plays a role in determining the alignment of the spine, shoulders, and skull. It is key to visualize samasthiti (even standing) in the sitting bones and then to generate equal balance on both sides of the pelvis. The seated pose *daṇḍāsana* (staff pose) is the samasthiti of the seated poses as it helps to orient and balance the two sides of the body.

PRACTICE

Moving from Your Pelvic Heels

This exploration involves minute articulation of the two pelvic hemispheres. It helps assess leg-length discrepancy and will indicate if one side of the pelvis is habitually pulled downward toward the heel (called downslip) or hiked upward toward the head (called upslip). The movement also gives the practitioner a distinct sense of the correlation between the heel of the foot and the heel of the sitting bone.

Lie on your back and allow your entire body to relax for several minutes. In keeping with the intention to build more somatic intelligence through sensing, scan your legs and inquire: Does one leg feel longer than the other? Does one leg rotate out more than the other? Before moving, place your fingertips on the bony landmarks of your anterior superior iliac spine (ASIS) at the front of your pelvis. Again inquire: Does one side of your pelvis push up toward the ceiling more than the other? Is one ilia hiked upward toward your head? Then with your foot flexed, push the heel of one foot away from your head while remaining passive in the other leg. Avoid bending your knee or lifting your leg off the floor. Flex your foot by pulling your toes toward your head and at the same time extend through your Achilles tendon, calf, and hamstring. Notice how the sitting bone of your extended leg scoots downward (away from your low back). Notice how the opposite ilium shifts upward toward your lumbar spine. Continue with this alternating movement of upslip and downslip. This offsetting of the ilia replicates the motion of the pelvis in walking. Notice how the sitting bone and the heel move together and assess whether one side of your pelvis moves with greater ease than the other side. Repeat fifteen to twenty times.

Uttānāsana and the Three Sets of Heels

This posture helps establish a clear polarity between the heels of the feet, the sitting bones of the pelvis, and the "heels" of the back of the skull. Aligning the calcanea and buttock bones brings a feeling of congruency and harmonious extension to your legs.

After practicing the supine exercise "Moving from Your Pelvic Heels," roll up and sit in daṇḍāsana (staff pose) with your legs straight out on the floor and your pelvis elevated on a one-inch-thick pad. As you descend your sitting bones, try to distribute your weight evenly between them. Notice if your buttock bones make equal contact with the pad. Then come to stand in tāḍāsana with your feet hip-width apart. Extend upward prior to folding forward into *uttānāsana* (intense forward bend) and place your hands on the floor with palms down. If you cannot reach, then prop your hands with several blocks, or hold on to a chair. Set your position so that each heel is aligned under the center of the corresponding sitting bone. Shift your thighbones forward in order to stand on the plumb line of your legs while raising your sitting bones upward. Allow your skull to release downward so that it suspends from the *cranial heels* at the back of your skull. Sense the internal alignment of the three sets of heels at your feet, pelvis, and skull. Notice in figure 2.4 the circular flow of the movement relative to the calcaneal, ischial, and cranial heels. Remain for two minutes, then move into downward dog and sense a similar orientation of the three sets of heels.

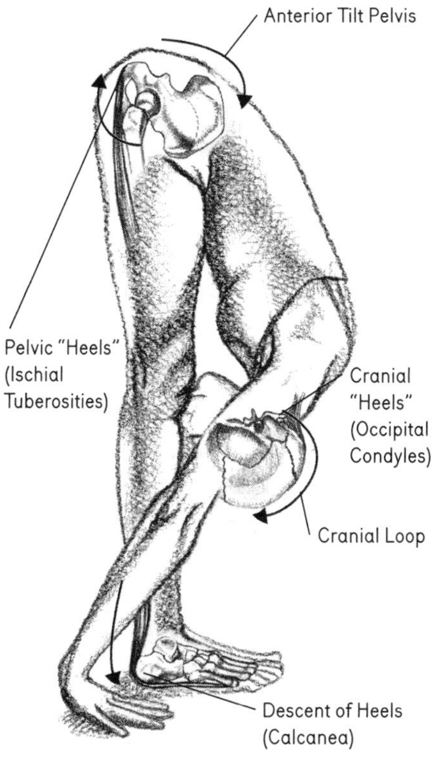

Figure 2.4 Uttānāsana and the Body's Three Sets of Heels

The Pelvic Diaphragm and Respiratory Diaphragm

A succession of horizontally oriented diaphragms partition and support various regions within the body (fig. 8.5). Each diaphragm can distend downward, contract inward, lift upward, and expand laterally. As we have seen, the plantar fascia, the thick fibrous webbing on the sole of the foot, is the first diaphragm; the pelvic diaphragm is the second. The pelvic floor is a perforated yet resilient muscular sling at the base of the pelvic cavity. Multiple slips of muscle comprise the sling, banded together in order to provide support for the pelvic organs.

Mūla Bandha

The pelvic floor has the capacity to alternately widen and narrow, then retract and drop. The net of musculature that forms the pelvic diaphragm does not act in isolation; its movements are linked to the muscles of the inner groins, hamstrings, buttocks, abdomen, and feet. It is important to remember that there is myofascial continuity between the muscles of the legs and the pelvic floor when learning mūla bandha. Internal lift at the spinal base is directly linked to, and follows upon, engaging the musculature of the legs. An isolated contraction of the pelvic floor is inadequate to disperse tension and bring a more full range of sensation and mobility to this area. Initially it is important to practice āsana in order to generate movement in the large muscles of the hips, inner groins, and upper thighs, that is, to work from the outside in. Once the clenched rigidity in the outlying areas of the exterior pelvis is reduced, then one can engage the more subtle articulations within the interior pelvis and pelvic floor.

An inordinate amount of strain may accumulate at the base of the spine within the first and second chakras. All too often the perineum is a receptacle for strain and can become a storehouse for repressed tension. When the body and mind are perceived to be under threat and there is gnawing or acute fear, the soft tissues of the perineum clamp in defensive reflex. This is particularly true in light of any trauma or violation in and around the pelvis. Combined postural and psychological pressure also build up in the hip joints, buttocks, low back, hamstrings, and groin. The flight-or-fight response typically shows up as constriction in the prime movers—the legs. Yet given that the perineum is supple, impressionable, and is the most yin tissue in the body, it is susceptible to strain and easily distressed.

One of the primary aims of practicing yoga is to encourage blood flow into the hips and pelvis, alternately saturating, flushing, and rinsing the structures within the pelvic bowl and lower spine. Proper circulation of fluids into the organs and glands combined with good neurological function can help regulate hormonal activity. One of the primary effects of a hip opener is vasodilation, which allows blood, lymph, and cellular fluid to bathe and nourish the tissues. Yoga postures together with the ḷift of mūlā bandha help change the pressure dynamics in and around the pelvic floor, thereby monitoring neurological and circulatory rhythms within the pelvic cavity. For example, in *vinyāsa* yoga practice, the perineum alternately expands and narrows. In the course of the sun salutation when doing cobra or *ūrdhva mukha śvānāsana* (upward-facing dog pose), the pelvic floor retracts. Conversely, in downward dog the pelvic floor releases and widens.

The Anatomy of the Pelvic Floor

The perineum is shaped like a diamond, with the anterior triangle housing the genitalia and the posterior triangle surrounding the anus. The anterior perineum is yin, for it contains the reproductive organs, and the back portion is yang, for it includes the base of the digestive tract, the root of the colon, and the anus. Each of these triangular muscular webbings can be engaged in isolation. A pulse of movement, a vibratory quiver, felt in the anterior triangle and specifically in the central tendon between the two triangles, is the essence of mūla bandha and correlates to the movement of kuṇḍalinī. Physiologically, isolating the sensory current within the anterior triangle is both subtle and elusive. Activating the bundle of muscle at the posterior triangle (including the anal sphincter muscles) is more available to voluntary control. Gripping the tailbone portion of the perineum is called *ashvinī mudrā* (named for the way the hindquarters of a horse grip when coming to a stop) and includes contraction of the cylindrical rings around the anus. Contracting and alternately expanding the anterior triangle is linked to the subtle body due to its effects on reproductive vitality and *ojas*, the body's most refined tissue (*dhātu*). Ojas refers to semen in the male body and the ovum in the female body, and their cyclical movements that are governed by hormonal rhythms within the brain. For men, anatomically controlling the anterior perineal triangle is linked to ejaculation control, an ability that is regarded in both Taoist and yoga practices to be the key to overall vitality. By yoking the anterior perineum, the pranic sheath within the body (*prāṇa-maya-kośa*) expands and is fortified. Control of the perineum is valuable generally, because as people age the contractile capacity of the urethra wanes and both men and women suffer from incontinence. Mūla bandha helps maintain the sphincter control necessary for timed urination.

PRACTICE

Mūla Bandha: Catch and Release for the Pelvic Floor

The following practice is a good way to engage mūla bandha without causing excessive constriction. Rather than a single contraction, it involves a series of pulsatory contractions of the pelvic floor. Sit in *siddhāsana* (accomplished pose) and place your heel (traditionally the left one) at the midpoint between the anus and genital (at the root of the scrotum for men and at the posterior margin of the vagina for women). This mechanical pressure helps soften rigidity within the pelvic floor and foster a parasympathetic response in the body. Lightly press against the central tendon of the perineum with your heel. The tendon will feel like a small bundle of knobby fibers the size of a small coin. Draw an inhalation down your spine into your perineum, making your breath a thin stream, like the smoke from an incense stick.

While seated in siddhāsana, align the center of your skull over the center of your pelvis. Be sure to release your jaw and tongue, as constriction in the mandible is often coupled with strain in the pelvic floor. Begin by relaxing the tissues in and around your pelvic floor. Take several long, slow breath strokes. Once your breath has settled, exhale deeply and, *at the end of the exhalation,* contract your perineum rhythmically in a set of seven pulses, in what amounts to a catch-and-release action. Then take a long inhalation, brushing your breath against your spine. Repeat five to ten times, and with each series of mini-contractions, sense the anal sphincter muscles engage. This results in grip around the tailbone. Generally it is best to avoid clenching the soft tissues around the tailbone, for binding at the coccyx restrains spinal motion. Attempt to bring the pulsating contractions to the anterior margin of your perineum so that you are pumping the musculature at the root of the genitalia. Feel the way the pulsing actions aid in suffusing blood flow into your pelvic floor and track any corresponding release that may take place around your jaw, ears, and skull. Following this exercise, sit quietly and breathe normally. Notice a feeling of levity and expansion in your spine, as if your spine is rising and spreading like a column of steam. Practice this technique for five minutes and then sit for another ten minutes with a full, soft diaphragmatic breath. Afterward lie in śavāsana to rest.

Pregnancy and the Pelvic Floor

The perineum is vulnerable to prolapse, due to the weight of collapsing organs, as a result of forced defecation, or from trauma during labor. During vaginal birth, descending pressures from the fetal cranium against the pelvic floor may cause the perineum to overstretch, tear, and lose contractile capacity. Following birth, the pelvic floor and the uterus may prolapse. This is due to the rigors and strain involved with downward abdominal force and laxity within the core structures of the pelvis and abdomen. Postdelivery, an episiotomy can also compromise the pelvic floor, leading to scar tissue and abnormal pulling within the musculature of the pelvic diaphragm.

A postnatal yoga practice helps to generate greater structural integrity to the pelvic diaphragm, as well as in the inner groins, hip rotator muscles, and abdomen. To prevent or minimize the likelihood of postpartum prolapse, women are advised to wait until the pelvic organs have returned to their pre-pregnancy size before returning to active practice. This can take up to two months after delivery. A protocol for postnatal yoga includes the harmonious coordination of mūla bandha and uḍḍīyāna bandha, in order to gently lift the pelvic organs and engage the pelvic floor muscles. Kegel exercises, which are similar to mūla bandha, are valuable prenatally and postnatally to tone, strengthen, and maintain pliability of the musculature within the pelvic diaphragm. Kegels, or mūla bandha specifically, help to fortify the bulbospongiosus muscle that weaves like an infinity symbol on the pelvic floor in the space between the coccyx and pubic bone.

The Bulbous Root and Coils of Kuṇḍalinī

The ancient yogis likened the body to a plant and the stabilizing structures of the tailbone and sacrum to roots. In the esoteric imagination of kuṇḍalinī yoga, the first chakra (mūlādhāra) is burrowed under the earth and resembles an underground bulb called a *kanda*. Embedded in darkness, the bioenergetics of the first chakra lie latent and unexpressed. Thus, the first chakra is of the earth, inseparable from it, and holds potential for growth.

The word *mūla* translates as root, source, or foundation. In the body it implies a root formation, a bundle, or a packet. If you have pulled out weeds from your garden, you may have noticed that a plant has not only one root but anchors into the earth via a cluster of root filaments. Thus, we could think of the mūlādhāra as a knotted mass. The root chakra is the radicle of the revered central channel of the body, a current whose deep pulse governs all autonomic functioning in the body. In the *Śiva Saṁhitā*, a text on the subtle energetics of haṭha yoga compiled in the seventeenth century, the mūlādhāra chakra is described this way:

> Two fingers above the rectum and two fingers below the *linga*, four fingers in width is a space like a bulbous root. Between this space is the yoni having its face towards the back: there dwells the goddess *Kuṇḍalinī*. It surrounds all the *nāḍīs*, and has three coils and a half; and catching its tail in its own mouth, it rests in the hole of the *suṣumnā*.[3]

The metaphor of the bulb, like the metaphor of the coiled serpent, suggests a force that is latent and full of potential. The kuṇḍalinī, related to the reptilian brain, is the creative source of all becoming.

Haṭha yoga looks to untangle the neurological and psychospiritual knot of this primal energy and direct it upward to the lungs, heart, and brain. Note how in the pose kandāsana (see fig. 2.2) the feet, placed on the navel, serve to propel the force of kuṇḍalinī up the spine.

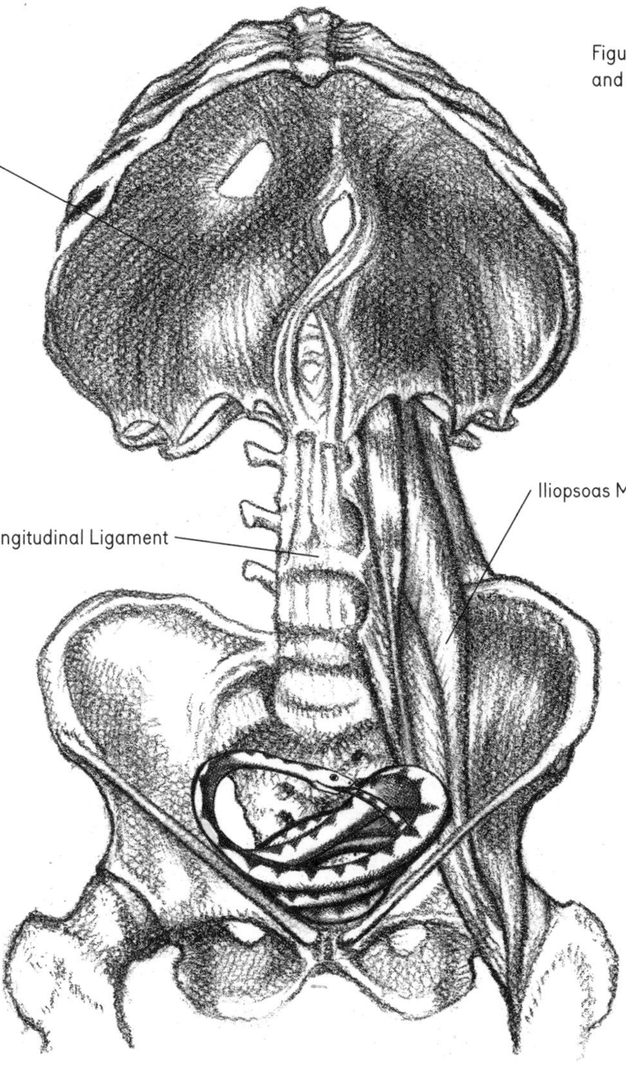

Figure 2.5 The Iliopsoas and the Lair of Kuṇḍalinī

Dreams, Kuṇḍalinī, and Control

In psychological terms, the unconscious is linked to the serpent at the base of the spine; the spiritual Self is entangled in the roots. States of yogic concentration (samādhi) reveal glimpses of the spirit Self buried in the underworld. The yoga tradition navigates this earthen darkness through dreams, visions, revelations, and myth. For years yogis have looked to sleep states and dream as means to delve into the unconscious. Both Freud and Jung's initial research on depth psychology included extensive investigation of dream content. Certain dream images and feelings in a dream suggest the depths of the lower chakras. The force of the mūlādhāra get dramatized in dreams as oceans, waterborne reptiles, dark forests, underwater caves, wells, catacombs, basements, and more.

Disentangling the knotted coils of the serpent goddess Kuṇḍalinī suggests loosening the locked power of the unconscious. This typically prompts a flood of inner sensation both sublime and terrible. The depth psyche holds sensations that are untenable to the ego. These sensations, related to kuṇḍalinī, are habitually sublimated and repressed due to the fact that their power and magnitude threaten the egoic self. Reflexes within the overarching ego attempt to control the power of the unconscious and defend itself from forces within the underworld. It wishes to keep the force of kuṇḍalinī concealed, inert, and incapacitated. Yogis look to do just the opposite. Through physiological and psychological technique, they aim to awaken or animate the reptilian force. This process is extremely difficult since the egoic self tenaciously adheres to its presumed position of authority and control.

In the subtle body, the coil of the kuṇḍalinī is dormant within the root cluster at the spinal base. This bulbous root mass is also called a *granthi* and refers to either a knotted bundle or the segmented joints on the shaft of a reed or cane. Recall that in the creation myth of the birth of the Native American Pueblo people, a cosmic stalk with segmented, chakra-like openings rises upward from the center of the earth. In the body, along the "stalk" of the spine beginning at the base, there are three main knots or psychic seals to be broken or decoded:

the *Brahma granthi* at the spinal base, the *Vishnu granthi* at the heart, and the *Śiva granthi* between the eyebrows.

In keeping with the analogy of the spine as a water plant, we can imagine a water lotus growing in a pool or lake, its stem dangling down to the depths and its root mass tethering it to the mud. This root system pumps nutrients upward to the leaves and flower, in the way that the tailbone works to pump a series of pulses—part liquid, part electric—through the spine. The earthbound mūlādhāra chakra is thus the fount for the origin of life. The gnarled root ball (kanda) is necessary to feed the flowers above, channeling its vitality into the spine, organs, and brain.

Sacred Geometry and the Mūlādhāra Chakra

In the architecture of the chakras, the geometric design associated with the mūlādhāra chakra is the square. The square is figured at the base because its shape implies stability and longevity. Throughout India, Nepal, and Tibet, the square is the architectural foundation for temples and stupas. The square establishes the temple firmly into the earth in the way that the mūlādhāra chakra anchors the spine. The square represents grounding, containment, and the source of creation.

Throughout the history of yoga discipline, sacred symbols called *yantras* depict the cosmic order of consciousness. They are devices to enhance meditative awareness and are guides to the psyche's interior. The outer frame of the yantra is a square. The square is the periphery, the doorway, whose openings enable progression from exterior to interior and from gross to subtle. It is a shape that both contains and supports. At the base of the spine, the four-sided square is the first threshold one must pass in order to gain access to the sacred interior (see figs. 2.6 and 7.5).

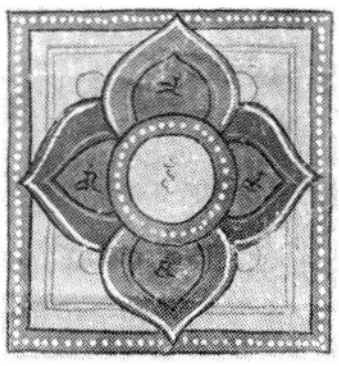

Figure 2.6 Square Yantra Mūlādhāra Chakra

In the way that the mūlādhāra is the first rung of the chakra system, the square is the entrance into the labyrinthine power grid of the yantra's interior. The peripheral square is gated. With doorways in the four cardinal directions, it allows entrance, but only to the one who has first abandoned the material and emotional obsessions that confine her.

Related to the configuration of the square, the first chakra is associated with the elephant. Like the weight of earth that embeds the mūlādhāra, the hefty elephant is the quintessential earthbound animal. Its strength, rootedness, passion, and intelligence suggest the vitality of the first chakra. In myths and rituals native to India, the enduring, steadfast, and bullish elephant transports *mahārājas* and *devas* atop its magnificent frame. In a similar way, the square-shaped sturdy mūlādhāra supports the celestial chakras at the top of the vertebral column.

On the Lotus Pad of Transcendental Wisdom

In Hindu and Buddhist iconography, the meditating yogi, absorbed in samādhi, is frequently depicted upon a throne of lotus petals. For instance, in the Buddhist tradition, there are innumerable representations of Shākyamuni Buddha; Mañjuśrī, the bodhisattva of wisdom; and Avalokiteśvara, the bodhisattva of compassion, seated in profound contemplation atop a floating lotus pad. These enlightened figures, made of bronze or brass, are gilded, lacquered, painted, and are typically adorned with semiprecious jewels. The sculptural figures rest on an ornamental flower base featuring lustrous petals of gold or white. Installed amid lotus petals, enlightened figures appear like carpels inside a blossoming flower.

The motif of the flower pedestal or underlying lotus pad suggests that the entire wisdom tradition stands on an enlightened base. In the evolution through the chakras, the lotus seat at the root chakra, comprised of four petals, bursts forth as the *sahasrāra chakra,* defined as the "thousand-petaled lotus" at the crown. In iconography depicting yogic wisdom, not only is the lotus pad a source of spiritual awakening but the lotus stalk too is considered to be a conduit for spiritual knowledge. For instance, Mañjuśrī is often depicted holding a delicate lotus stem in one hand. At the apex of the stem blooms the great text of Mahāyāna Buddhism, the *Heart Sutra of Transcendental Wisdom* (*Prajñāpāramitā Sūtra*).

Drawing Inward—The Tortoise and the Path of Absorption

In the internal arts of yoga and qigong, a delicate yet profound activation of the perineal fibers animates the subtle body. One of the classical aims of mūla bandha for yogic practitioners (primarily men) was to sublimate the sexual current and direct its current inward. This enabled monks and sadhus to convert the potent biological force situated in the pelvis into the breath of spirit located in the heart.

In classical haṭha yoga, interiority is thought to animate prāṇa, increase physical vitality, and enable consciousness to absorb into itself. Of all creatures, the turtle best exemplifies this process of involution and absorption. Together with the serpent, the turtle is a reptile prized in the yoga tradition for its innate wisdom and longevity (giant tortoises are known to have lived for 185 years). Like the kuṇḍalinī, the turtle is stationed at the base of the spine.

The turtle (*kūrma*) has a unique capacity to retract its limbs and its head. For the yogi, this remarkable achievement symbolizes a concentration of both mental and physical energies away from worldly endeavors. Introversion is a means not only to safeguard the precious life-force but to fortify the mind and make it one-pointed. In the Bhagavad Gītā, Kṛṣṇa counsels the warrior Arjuna on the battlefield, "When one completely withdraws the sensory organs from outside stimuli, just as a tortoise pulls its limbs into its shell, one becomes established in wisdom."[4]

Suggested here is the yogic practice of *pratyāhāra*, internalization of the sensory awareness, the fifth limb of Patañjali's Aṣṭāṅga Yoga path.[5] We will investigate the dynamics of pratyāhāra in detail in chapter 8. Pratyāhāra not only involves turning the eyes, ears, tongue, and nostrils inward but includes harnessing the libidinal charge located in the pelvic floor and reproductive center. Mūla bandha protects, clarifies, and refines the libidinal force and, like an internal dynamo, tantalizes and enlivens the reptilian power. A steady surge of kuṇḍalinī in the subtle body heightens and expands sensitivity, energizes the spine, expands breathing, and concentrates the mind.

Figure 2.7 The Turtle Pose and the Interiority of Sensory Awareness

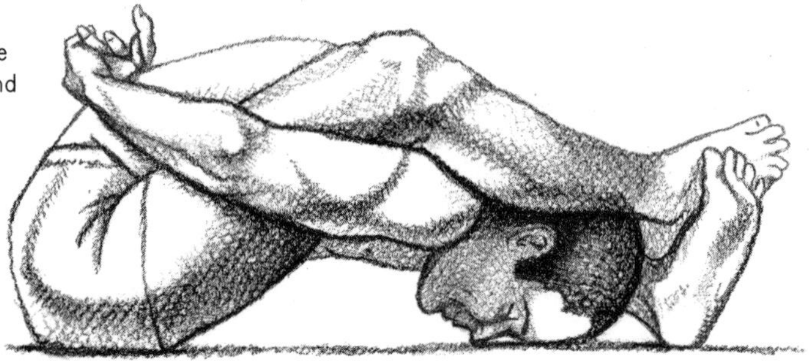

Kurmāsana (turtle pose) conveys a similar withdrawal of the senses, for the head is drawn inside while the hands and feet latch, forming a kind of secure stronghold or barricade. The spine is rounded in the shape of a turtle's protective shell (fig. 2.7). All forward bends support interiority of the sensory organs, yet kurmāsana involves such profound spinal flexion that it can be considered an extreme form of introverting.

The Turtle That Upholds the World

The snake and turtle are prominently featured in Hindu creation myths, particularly in the story of "The Churning of the Ocean of Milk," one of the most provocative and delightful myths describing the origin of life. The story goes something like this: according to legend, the world is motionless, in a deep sleep (*yoga nidrā*) and nothing stirs. There is no life, no pulse, no wind, no prāṇa. At the bottom of this vast sea, the kūrma resides, supporting everything. It has mounted on its back the first landmass, Mount Meru, rising straight up in the water like a cosmic spinal column, the *Śiva linga*, the procreative staff of life. A magnificent snake is coiled around the base of the mountain like a giant cord. Yet nothing stirs, there is no movement of life until the gods and demons, oppositional forces of good and evil, life and death, partake in a cosmic tug of war. The gods take one end of the serpent and the demons take hold of the other end and they pull, with great enduring vigor. As they compete, the serpent, coiled around the mountain, begins to revolve (conjuring the awakening of kuṇḍalinī), and all of life is generated from the ripples and fluctuations caused by its spin.

This myth is reminiscent of the chore of churning milk into butter via a blender-like apparatus, a daily task in Indian village life for centuries. This churning represents alchemical shifts, both physiological and spiritual, that take place through yogic tapas. In the way that the archetypal pillar in the cosmic ocean is spun through force, haṭha yoga churns the spine through āsana. Yoga poses, as in "The Churning of the Ocean of Milk," provide oppositional movements fraught with dynamic tension, and so generate creative flow.

Like the pelvis that supports the spine, the turtle supports the primeval mountain, Mount Meru on its back, the world's central axis. Thus, the figure of the turtle is integral to the first chakra, the mūlādhāra. Cosmologically, its steadfast presence upholds all of creation.

It is interesting to note that in Native American folklore, especially in various Northeastern tribes such as the Iroquois and Algonquin, the turtle plays a similar role in mythology as the bearer of the North American landmass. Akin to myths from India (and the book of Genesis), at the beginning of time all was water, leaving no solid ground upon which living beings could stand and take refuge. In the Haudenosaunee (Iroquois) creation story, a woman falls from the great sky world, and as she descends toward the water, animal beings confer as to how to help her. A prodigious turtle (with the help of a trustworthy muskrat) volunteers to offer his shell as she lands. Thus, the back of the turtle becomes the host or *island* for the North American continent and the refuge for all people. For this reason the Iroquois imagined their native landmass to be propped atop the back of a turtle and thus called North America, Turtle Island.

The Central Channels of Life

In traditional Chinese medicine there are two central meridians that travel between the pelvic floor and the skull, the Conception Vessel (*Ren mai*) and the Governing Vessel (*Du mai*). The Conception Vessel is the yin channel, oriented on the front body, while the yang channel, the Governing Vessel, extends up the back of the body. The Conception and Governing Vessels have auxiliary pathways that directly

Figure 2.8 Central Channels and the Deep Life-Force

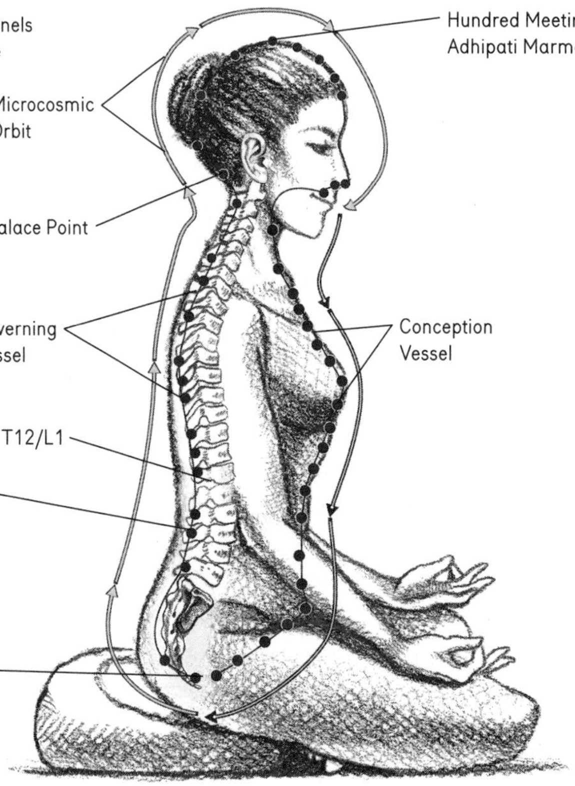

penetrate the spinal column. Both of these meridians have their source in the mūlādhāra chakra, the root of the body, within the pelvic floor. At the top of the spine they come together in the upper palate. The connection of the two meridians, from the center of the pelvic floor to the mid-palate, is known as the Microcosmic Orbit.

In meridian theory, the nadir of the body is considered to be the most yin (soft, diffuse, receptive, dark, lunar, yielding, slow, and watery) while the apex of the skull is thought to be the most yang point in the body (fast, hard, solid, bright, solar, masculine, and focused). In the Taoist tradition, the Conception and Governing Vessels link opposite yet complementary forces—Heaven and Earth, midday and midnight, the dynamic and the receptive, and male and female. Like the interpenetrating halves of the symbol for the Tao, the dynamic tension between yin and yang channels are responsible for all physiological function.

In Taoist practice it is essential to descend the breath into the sea of vitality at the depth of the spine (the lower *dan tian*) between the navel and the pelvic floor. Circulating the prāṇa in and through the pelvis enlivens the meridian pathways that link upward to the skull (fig. 2.8).

PRACTICE

From Coccyx to Crown: Sensing the Polarity of Yin and Yang

This meditation serves to bring awareness to the extreme ends of the spine, from the lowest tip of the coccyx to the very crown of the skull. This practice brings to light how the first chakra, the mūlādhāra chakra, and the seventh chakra, the sahasrāra chakra, are remotely paired (see fig. 7.5). In Taoist practice, to be fully human means to balance between heaven (at the top of the skull) and earth (at the pelvic diaphragm). This exercise serves to harmonize the upward-moving yang and downward-flowing yin while circulating the prāṇa within the Microcosmic Orbit of the body. The focus is to descend the energy of the brain to the base while simultaneously lifting upward from the sea of vitality in the lower pelvic region.

Assume a comfortable seated pose and orient the crown of your head directly over your pelvis. Settle into a soft and resonant breath. Place the pad of the middle finger of one hand at the tip of your coccyx and the pad of the middle finger of your other hand on the crown of your head. Sense the extreme ends of your spinal column and imagine the two points sharing a kind of magnetic resonance. Sense the vibrational pulse between your two fingers at the extreme ends of your spine. At the same time place the tip of your tongue to the roof of your mouth, where the Conception and Governing Vessels complete an internal circuit, the Microcosmic Orbit (see fig. 2.8).

Release your fingertip contact at the tailbone and crown and let your hands rest on your thighs. Now with soft and steady breathing, descend your breath into your navel area. Concentrate on expanding your inhale into the lowest part of your abdominal balloon, between your navel and your pelvic floor. This is a downward movement. Then focus the prāṇa in your spine and move upward from your tailbone to your kidneys at the point where the twelfth thoracic vertebra and first lumbar vertebra meet (T12 and L1). Continue to draw a steady stream upward along the back of your spine (through the Governing Vessel) to the area of your brain stem. This upward movement is best done on exhalation. Then lift the back of your skull gently upward and sense an ascending movement to the crown of your head. The apex of the cranium is the Hundred Meeting Point where all meridians in the body converge. Called the Mountain of Heaven in traditional Chinese medicine (*Du 20*), this point is thought to pacify any rising winds that move upward into the head. Now inhale down the front of your body, visualizing the breath's descent from your forehead over your face, neck, sternum, and abdomen down to your navel center where you started the circuit. This descending movement follows the path of the Conception Vessel. Continue to create a slow circular, orbiting loop with your breath. Stay for ten to fifteen minutes.

Baddha Koṇāsana in Śīrṣāsana

Of all yoga postures śīrṣāsana, the headstand, helps to establish a connection between the yang center at the top skull and the most yin point at the tailbone. An intermediate yoga posture, headstand inverts the spine so the nadir becomes the crown and the crown the nadir. It flips the yin and yang polarity, so that the apex of the skull becomes the lowest and most yin (receptive) point in the body. This soothes and calms the nerves of the brain and sensory organs.

Assume śīrṣāsana (headstand), resting your weight on a point an inch or so in front of the crown of your head. Be sure to firmly press your forearms to the floor and raise your shoulders. Avoid compression of your neck and skull by actively raising your legs. Stretch the central channel of your inside leg and actively stretch the skin on the soles of your feet. Once in the pose, remain with legs extended for a minute, then move your feet into baddha koṇāsana (bound angle pose). Press your heels together and actively raise your tailbone. Do not clench or narrow your perineum but widen it. In headstand, what is generally the most yin point of the body, at the tip of the coccyx, becomes active and dynamic (yang) as it assumes the role of pinnacle of the spine. Align your pelvis directly over your skull so that the epicenter of your perineum balances above the top of your skull. Avoid aligning your trunk too far forward or backward, thereby harmonizing the Conception Vessel on the front of your body with the Governing Vessel in the back.

If you are unable to perform a headstand, do downward-facing dog pose with your head supported by a bolster and rest the weight of your head an inch or two anterior to the crown of your head. In downward dog, set your feet as wide as your mat in order to broaden your perineum and stretch the tissues around your tailbone. After headstand follow with shoulderstand in order to release any compression around your neck.

Getting to the Root

In many regards, the discipline of yoga involves getting to the root. In this chapter we have established how the base of the spine and pelvic floor serve as roots for the entire body. The concept of the root is so central to yoga theory and practice that we talk about "root teachers," "root texts," and in Sankhya philosophy refer to the root of the manifest world (*mūlaprakṛti*). We have seen how the root support (mūlādhāra) is the origin of the chakra system relating to the body's innermost biological rhythms. Spiritual transformation does not simply require an upward movement; rather, it is paramount that one tap into the depths. This enables not only connection to the structures at the base of the spine but connection to the root of the breath (*prāṇamūla*) and to the very source of consciousness (*cittamūlā*). In the next chapter we continue this plummet to the depths by exploring the centerpiece of the pelvis, the sacred sacrum.

3

THE SACRED SACRUM

The Watery Realm of the Lower Spine

Just as a blue lotus blossom,
a red or white lotus blossom,
is born and grows in water,
but comes out of water
and is not attached to water,
the Tathāgata (Buddha) is born
and grows in the world,
comes out of the world,
and is not attached to the world.[1]

—The Middle Way Discourses of the Buddha

As we begin our trek up the spine from the subterranean depths of the pelvis, we climb a short distance and arrive at the cave of the sacrum, a grotto of latent power and abode of the water chakra. The sacrum plays a vital role in the yoga body, both anatomically as the substratum of the spine and in the mystical yoga tradition as a repository for reptilian power. Structurally the sacrum is considered to be the keystone of the pelvis for it transfers kinetic forces from the legs to the spine. The sacrum orients movement of all kinds; all yoga poses achieve stability and somatic integration via the bearing that the sacrum provides. In the subtle body, the cavernous shape of the anterior sacrum is the cache of the slumbering omnipotent serpent goddess, kuṇḍalinī, who is awakened through physical discipline and psychic concentration.

The Crux of the Sacrum

As the crux of the entire vertebral column, the sacral position is unique; it plays two roles, one part pelvis and one part spine. Within the pelvis, it plays a pivotal role as centerpiece at the back of the pelvis, permitting movement through the sacroiliac (SI) joints (see fig. 2.1). As part of the spine, it forms the base of the spine and acts like a rudder, helping to stabilize and steer the entire vertebral column. Equilibrium within the sacrum is critical for orienting and aligning all twenty-four bones of the spine plus the skull.

We could imagine how the spine is like a cairn of stones stacked on the side of a hiking trail. The cairn is an archaic symbol used throughout history to orient and determine location. When constructing a cairn, the placement of the very first stone establishes the balance for all other stones in the vertical architecture. Similarly, the structural alignment of the sacrum and tailbone reinforces support for all the other vertebrae in the column.

Another salient architectural design that describes the central role of the sacrum is that of the Roman arch. In the Roman arch, the keystone at the top upholds the weight of the two vaulted sides. Similarly, the sacrum, wedged between the two sides of the pelvis, braces the entire spine-pelvis complex. Kinetic forces passing through the sacrum are transferred to the right and left wings of the pelvis (the ilia). In this way the sacrum is the point of convergence between the right and left sides of the body, helping to equalize forces that are transmitted up through the legs (fig. 3.1).

Figure 3.1 Roman Arch and the Keystone of the Sacrum

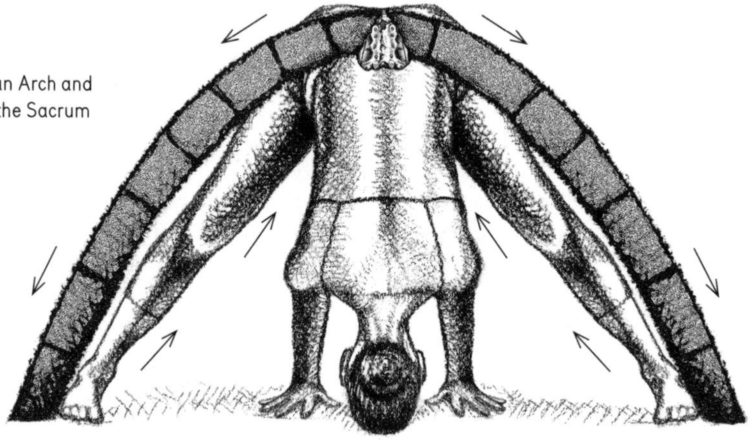

The Holy Bone

The sacrum is the *holy bone* in more ways than one. First, it is the sacrosanct bone of the body's physical structure. The ancient Greeks deemed the sacrum holy because they considered it to be the one bone in the body that never decomposed. This idea may have had its origins in the fact that the sacrum is one of the strongest bones in the body, composed of dense, compact cortical tissue. The central location of the sacrum at the base of the spine means that equilibrium within the sacrum is critical and has associations with the exquisite nectar of the gods, amṛta, the famed source of immortality.

It is also holy because it is literally pocked with holes, or foramina. Apertures in the sacral bone provide openings for nerve roots exiting the spine—nerve tracts that travel into the pelvis and further down the leg (fig. 3.2). These perforations not only permit nerves to travel; they lend a quality of lightness to the sacrum. The foramina afford the sacrum suspension and give it an aerodynamic character, making possible arabesques in classical ballet or the loft of *bakāsana,* the crane pose, in yoga.

As the first chakra, the mūlādhāra chakra, pertains to the earth element, the second chakra, the *svādhiṣhṭhāna chakra,* is associated with water. We can think of the sacrum containing a fluid vitality, akin to

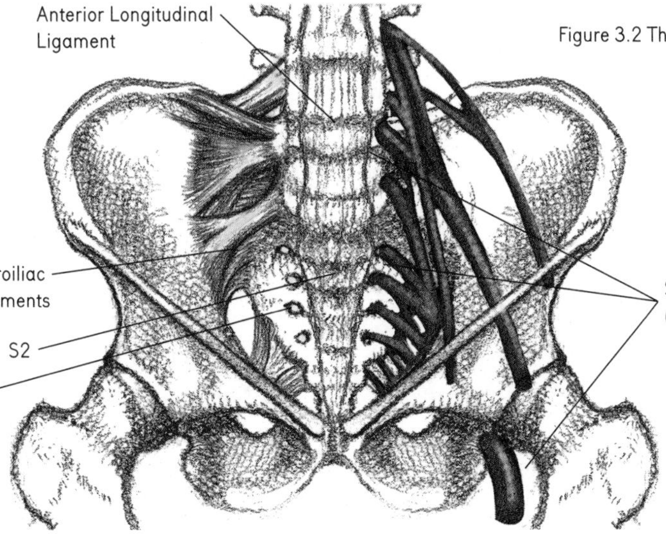

Figure 3.2 The Sacral Plexus

the dark and watery realm at the base of a well shaft. The watery realm of the sacrum has anatomical associations with the bladder, a storage tank for fluid located just anterior to the sacrum; the ureters, which siphon excess water from the kidneys and trail down to the bladder; and the large intestine, which absorbs water prior to elimination and attaches directly to the front of the sacrum.

The sacrum is also linked to the fluid realm due to its role as a hydraulic pump driving cerebrospinal fluid (CSF) up and down the spinal cord. The cerebrospinal fluid, one of the most rarefied fluids in the body, bathes the brain and spinal nerves. Its flow is generated in part by the rhythmic contractions and expansions of the sacral bone.

Critical for the subtle body, the fluid makeup of the sacral plexus includes the reproductive organs: the uterus, ovaries, testes, and seminal ducts, all of which are associated with the second chakra. In the female body the uterus is attached to the sacrum by the uterosacral ligament. Yoga, Āyurveda, and qigong look to support the fluid vitality within the reproductive organs: the seminal fluid in males and the uterine blood and ovarian fluid in females. In women, this fluid vitality depends in part on a regular and harmonious menstrual cycle. The essential vitality of the reproductive cycle is referred to in Sanskrit as *ojas* and has real influence over the subtle body. Ojas is linked to the body's immunity and, when radiant, provides the body with physical luster, potency, magnetism, and longevity. Ojas not only is the tissue of the procreative force but contains a divine spark that animates and sustains prāṇa.

In Search of the Dragon and Reptilian Power

Depiction of a great libidinous reptile lurking in the depths is not unique to haṭha yoga. An all-powerful, semi-aquatic reptile is also found in Chinese lore. In China the dragon is given high status, celebrated for its invincibility and power. The dragon is the quintessential metaphor for longevity, steadfastness, and endurance. Its presence is auspicious, as it grants vitality, might, and good fortune. Like the sacral chakra that is governed by the water element, in China the dragon is a creature that presides over watery realms—lakes, oceans, and rivers.

In tales from the Far East and in Western mythology, the dragon is associated with fame, wealth, and physical prowess. Within the dragon's domain are heaps of riches—jade, emeralds, rubies, and gold coins. A common motif in Chinese iconography is that of the well-endowed dragon clenching a jewel, reluctant to let it go. Clamped between its jaws or held fast under its chin, the jewel is carefully guarded. In the way that the dragon clenches a pearl or jade stone in its mandibular clutches, constriction in the sacrum is often coupled with jaw strain. Physical, emotional, and psychological tensions conspire, rendering sacral-mandibular tension intractable.

This reptilian force is at once enlightening and potentially destructive. John Woodruffe coined the term "the Serpent Power" in his 1920 exposé on the kuṇḍalinī chakra system. The power of the reptile is subliminal, just beyond the scope of cognition and outside of conscious control. Harbored in the spinal depths within the autonomic nervous system, this primal and instinctual life governs our essential biorhythms, affecting breathing, hormonal firing, and states of arousal and rest. Thoughts, moods, and patterns of behavior stem from the coercive power (śakti) of this underlying force, and so it is the yogi's prerogative to rouse, vivify, and tame the kuṇḍalinī. Given its pervasive affect on the body, the reptilian instinct must be approached carefully. For this reason, many yoga texts caution against animating the serpent power without the guidance of an accomplished teacher.

Āsana, *prāṇāyāma* (retaining the breath), and the precise upward lift of the bandhas generate profound neurological shifts in the body. Yoga discipline emphasizes physical movements to trigger change in the autonomic nervous system, which controls the organs, glands, and smooth muscle of the body. Neuromuscular and neuroglandular shifts can awaken both physical and spiritual forces that are otherwise shut down, blocked, or distorted.

For millennia, shamanic practices from around the globe have targeted shifts within the autonomic nervous system. For example, Amazonian tribes conduct ceremonial rituals for healing and psychospiritual transformation by imbibing a psychoactive decoction of plant vines. The ayahuasca tea rituals affect the reptilian brain and kuṇḍalinī, as well as the vagus nerve that innervates the heart and digestive organs. The enchanting affects of ayahuasca taken as a ritual brew work in tandem with music and singing to produce spiritual visions and heal the subtle body.

That the kuṇḍalinī can be made spellbound is reflected in the magic of the snake charmer. A classic exhibition from India, depicted in scenes from Rudyard Kipling and today's Bollywood films, reveals a cobra being cajoled from the shadows of a wicker basket, rising mysteriously into the air, entranced by the high-pitched sound of a flute. This kind of trance points to how the raw, "primitive," or reptilian side of the nervous system can be awakened through delight and fascination. Similarily in the aesthetic arts of India, deep sentiment (*bhava*) is evoked via poetry, music (rāga), and dance in order to awaken feeling (tremors, tingles, quivers, and so forth) in the subtle body. In any case, whether by force or charm, the migration of this interior force begins with a loosening of the knotted constrictions within the spinal depths, prompting an ascending flow through the central channel of the spine.

The Crocodile and the Mythological Makara

The animal associated with the sacral chakra in the esoteric yoga tradition is the crocodile. Crocodiles are some of the most ancient creatures on the planet; fossil records show the oldest crocodile lived 240 million years ago in the Jurassic period. The potency of the second chakra is linked to this magnificent reptile because of its magnetism, brute force, sexual power, indomitable jaws, and side-to-side serpentine motion. In Hindu mythology and in the classic haṭha yoga text the Ṣaṭ Chakra Nirūpaṇa the crocodile appears as the *makara*, an imaginary creature akin to a sea dragon. It is a hybrid creature—half terrestial, half aquatic—that presides over the waters of the body. The makara could be said to govern all muscular activity within the pelvis and all internal and external secretions of the reproductive organs.

The makara serves as sentinel to sacred temples, deterring the insincere pilgrim. On temple facades throughout India the makara is depicted on perimeter panel walls. In the mythos of the body, it guards the opening to the spine at the cave of the sacrum and so must be contended with in order to gain entrance to the interior.

We can imagine the makara in the role as bearer of the vital waters. In Hindu iconography, the makara is host to the great river goddess Ganga and transports her on its back. Thus, the reptilian power of the makara upholds, sustains, and animates the fluid realm.

The Sacrum as the Center of Gravity

I like to think of the sacrum as the computer chip to the buttocks, legs, and feet because it is the nexus for the many nerve tracts that traverse the pelvis into the legs. In this regard we can imagine how the "intelligence" of the legs is governed by operations within the sacrum. The largest of these tracts is the sciatic nerve, a *mahā nāḍī* that has extensive communication with the leg and foot. The sciatic nerve is a bundle of nerve roots that emerges through the sciatic archway of the lower pelvis (see fig 3.2). Too large to exit only one segment of the spine, it emerges from the lower lumbar vertebrae and sacrum (the fourth lumbar vertebra through the third sacral segment), before it transits down into the leg. Given that the cluster of nerves emerging from the sacrum is so extensive, it is valuable to stretch and create space within the sacrum to allow for uninhibited neurological flow.

Most anatomists agree that the second sacral segment (S2) is the body's center of gravity. Not only is the sacrum the hub of the physical self, but it too is invested with the energy of the psyche. This is reflected in the name of the sacral chakra in Sanskrit, the svādhiṣṭhāna chakra. The prefix *sva* means "self," one's own, and *ṣṭhāna* suggests that which is established, stable, or secure. Thus, the sacrum, which is the quintessential bone of the svādiṣṭhāna chakra, implies self-possession or psychosomatic poise.

Structurally the sacrum plays a critical role in movement. Without a firm sense of center within the sacrum, the professional figure skater could not spin and leap, nor could the ballerina do a grand jeté across the stage. In yoga poses such as *piñca mayurāsana* (peacock pose) and *ūrdhva dhanurāsana* (upward bow pose), the sacrum within the pelvic girdle is the fulcrum for lift, levity, and balance. Having an established center of gravity in the sacrum is not only a resource for physical balance within the musculoskeletal structure; it is critical for helping to regulate neural, digestive, and endocrine function.

When we say that someone is "out of their center," we really mean to say that they have temporarily lost connection to their sacrum. When a body is rife with stress, a felt sense of equilibrium is lost and feelings of agitation creep upward (or sometimes fly upward in the face of real threat) and lodge in the solar plexus, shoulders, or neck. Emotional upheaval and repeated cycles of fear and irritability can divorce people from their own foundation. Yoga, tai chi, and qigong help students become grounded in their sacrum and thereby maintain a low center of gravity. Standing poses like triangle pose, flank pose, and the warrior poses provide stability and resiliency to the sacrum. A cultivated low center of gravity has a settling effect on the prānic body. In the meditative traditions when the chi or prāṇa pools in the sacral center, a calm alertness pervades the entire body.

PRACTICE

Setting the Keystone of the Sacrum

If the sacrum is a holy bone enshrined in the temple of the pelvis, then the legs are pillars that lead directly into the temple. In this guided standing pose, imagine the sacrum to be the keystone that unites the pillars of the legs.

Stand in *prasārita pādottānāsana* (wide-angle forward fold pose) so that your feet are three to four feet apart. Be sure that one foot is not forward of the other. Angle your feet slightly inward and press down the outer edges of your heels. The entire bank of your outer foot should anchor firmly into the floor. From the outer margin of your hip to your outer heels extend downward into the floor. Simultaneously raise the inner shaft of your leg from the inner arches of your feet to the top innermost groins. Lift the quadricep muscles at the front of your thighs in order to elongate your hamstrings (see fig 3.1).

Imagine your sacrum to be like the keystone at the top of a Roman arch. Visualize and feel the way the bony struts of your legs and pelvis act to stabilize your sacrum. From your outer right sacroiliac joint, extend down to your right heel, and from your outer left SI joint, extend down to your left heel. At the same time, widen your sacrum by rotating your thighs inward. Sense and feel the widening of both your posterior sacrum and the concave surface of your anterior sacrum where the bladder, colon, and reproductive organs are located. Firm your outer hip sockets (as you did in the Christmas tree technique described in chapter 2). This will help to secure your sacrum. Stay for two minutes.

Play in the Sacroiliac Joint

Achieving fluid movement within the sacrum is one of the primary aims of any practice in the internal arts, for if the sacrum becomes fixed, spinal motion from the sacrum to the skull will be restrained. As people age it is common for the sacroiliac joints to jam shut, especially in men, given their heavier build. As a consequence, the SI ligaments lose "play" as they become less pliable. If a sixty-year-old man shows up in a yoga class and is asked to step forward into a lunge, it may be arduous and cumbersome. He may have to manually lift his own leg and set it forward. This is indicative of adhesions within the fibrocartilage of his SI joint and may suggest partial fusion within the joint. Cadaver studies reveal that the SI joint ossifies for a significant portion of the population by the end of life.[2] The gait of someone who has a sacroiliac fixation appears wooden, and the leg, ilium, and sacrum swing forward as a single unit. Without give, play, or adaptability in the SI joints, the legs do not swing but appear to shuffle when walking.

The sacrum attaches firmly to the pelvis by way of resilient ligaments—ropy, sinewy structures that bear the weight of the entire spine and torso. (Notice the posterior sacroiliac joint ligaments in fig. 2.1 and the anterior sacroiliac joint ligaments in fig. 3.2.) Ideally, the right and left sides of the sacrum bear weight congruently in standing, sitting, and walking. However, due to repetitive strain or trauma, the ligaments on one side of the sacrum may become too taut (or too lax), potentially causing dysfunction in the sacroiliac joint. This is often coupled with unilateral muscular tension in the piriformis and gluteal muscles of the hip region.

A skilled osteopath, physical therapist, or chiropractor can identify sacroiliac restrictions and manually reset them. A sequence of yoga poses such as triangle pose, flank pose, half moon pose, cow pose, and *kapotāsana* (pigeon pose) take the ilia and sacrum through a range of possible movements (loosely coined "hip openers") that help maintain optimal stability of the sacroiliac joint.

PRACTICE

Freeing the Sacroiliac Joint

The aim of this practice is to isolate the movement of the pelvis one side at a time *relative to the sacrum* and test the range of motion within the sacroiliac ligaments. Isolating the movement of one pelvic hemisphere is a challenge. While seemingly simple, you may find it hard to individuate the following movements. Proceed slowly and gently and sense any regional asymmetries or holding patterns in your SI joints.

There are eight possible ways the ilium moves *relative to the sacrum*: upslip, when the ilium slides upward; downslip, when the ilium slides downward; outflare, when the ilium rotates outward; inflare, when the ilium rotates inward; anterior shift, when the ilium pushes forward; posterior shift, when the ilium pushes backward; anterior tilt, when the ilium rocks forward; and posterior tilt, when the ilium rocks backward.

Begin by lying on your back and allowing your entire body to relax. The entire sequence is done from the supine position. Remember that all movements should be done slowly and without excessive force. The soft, slow repetition of the movements helps to mobilize the sacrum and realign tensions within the sacroiliac joints.

PRACTICE

Upslip and Downslip

You will remember this movement from chapter 2, previously done to synchronize the heel and sitting bone. Push out through the heel of your right leg while remaining passive in the left. Slide the right ilium toward your heel and away from your sacrum. This is called downslip of the ilium. At the same time, notice how your opposite ilium slides upward toward your lower back. This is called upslip of the ilium. Stretch both legs out and release all holding. Repeat six to seven times, alternating sides.

PRACTICE

Outflare and Inflare

Bend your knees, place the soles of your feet on the floor, and take your right knee out to the side, like the bent knee position in tree pose. Keep your left knee vertical. This is outflare of the right ilium. Bring your right knee vertical and repeat the movement on your left side. Do the movement six to seven times, alternating side to side.

Now set your feet wider apart, keeping your knees bent. Swing your right knee toward your left foot by raising your right hip four to six inches off the floor; keep your left knee vertical. At the same time, arch your lower back. This is inflare of the right side of the pelvis. Repeat on the left side and again alternate the movement between your right and left sides six to seven times. Stretch both legs out and release any holding.

PRACTICE

Anterior and Posterior Shift

Bend your knees again and set your feet hip-width apart. Isolate movement into the right side of your pelvis by pressing the back of your right ilium into the floor. This is a posterior shift of the ilium on the right side. Notice that at the same time, your left ilium is drawn slightly upward toward the ceiling; this is anterior shift of the pelvis. Come back to center, then press your left ilium into the floor as you shift your right ilium toward the ceiling. These shifts are small and subtle and difficult to feel. Sense the slight movement in your sacroiliac ligaments as you alternately "walk" or "step" one ilium at a time into the floor. Alternate sides and repeat six to seven times. Stretch both legs out and release any holding.

PRACTICE

Posterior and Anterior Tilt

Bend your knees again and set your feet hip-width apart. The following movement replicates the motion of the ilia when walking. Draw your right knee toward your chest by lifting your foot six to ten inches off the floor. This is a posterior tilt of the right pelvic hemisphere. Simultaneously, slide your left thighbone away from your head, as if your left knee is lunging forward to press an imaginary button. Arch your lower back as you do the movement. This is anterior tilt of the left side of the pelvis. Repeat on your other side. This movement is like rotating a Rubik's Cube by turning one side of the cube toward you while rotating the opposite side away from you. Feel the opposing action within your right and left SI joints as you simultaneously rock one pelvic hemisphere into anterior tilt and the other into posterior tilt. Repeat six to seven times. Stretch both legs out and release all holding.

The sacrum bears the burden of the spinal column's weight. Just above the sacrum is the fifth and last lumbar vertebra (L5), and between L5 and the sacrum is a fluid-filled fibrocartilaginous disk. At the lower end of the spinal column, the supporting structures are prone to compression (fig. 3.3, Model A). Due to load-bearing forces set upon the lumbosacral hinge, it is common for the disk between L5 and the first sacral segment (S1) to degenerate, such that the disk ruptures and the nerves impinge. Most people lose some loft or buoyancy in the disks of the lower lumbar spine as they age. Yoga poses, when done carefully and in proper sequence, can help to stave off and counter these compressive forces.

Figure 3.3 Slumpasana and the Lower Spine

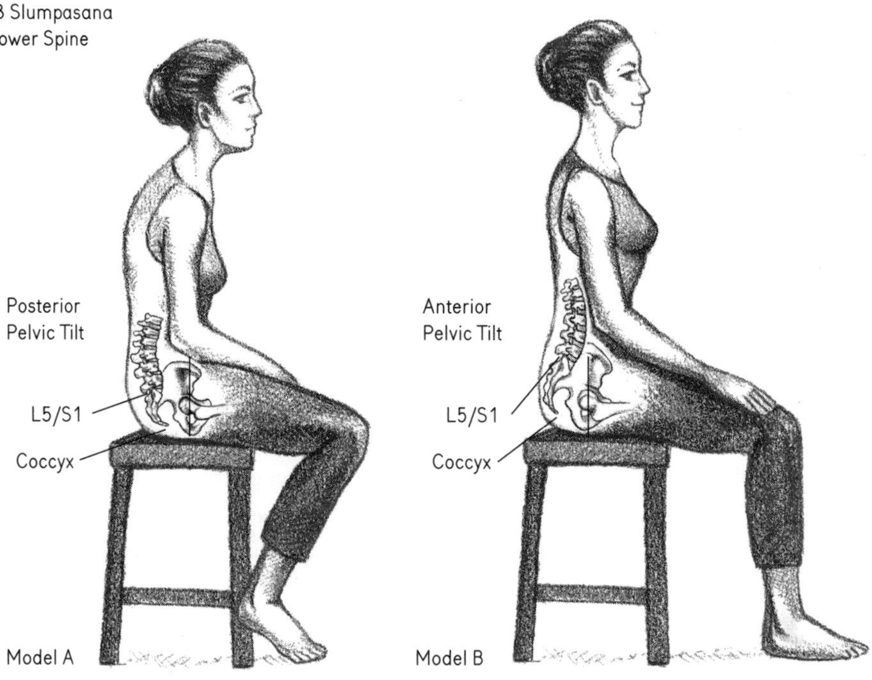

The Hazards of Slumpasana

When seated, posterior tilt of the pelvis involves a downward incline of the sacrum and collapse in the lower back. I think of this posterior droop as "slumpasana," a position that unfortunately gets held for hours and hours a day. Due to sitting for long periods of time, the lumbar spine loses its integrity and concave shape. This can be ruinous to the entire spine, as the lumbar spine plays a vital role in support. The lumbar vertebrae are stout, compact bones at the base of the spine, reinforced by powerful paraspinal muscles. When the lumbar capsizes backward, people lose the foundational support for their spine and trunk. When we say people are weak or "spineless" and do not have backbone, we are really saying that the stature within their lower back has fallen.

When the lumbar spine chronically collapses backward and downward, the fluid-filled, doughnut-shaped intervertebral disks that give the spine its characteristic buoyancy are compressed. Due to the backward slump of the spine, the disks become compacted and displace toward the back of the body. People with a history of posterior disk compression are vulnerable to the disk "slipping," protruding, or herniating during movements as simple as reaching down to pick up a toothbrush. *Bhujaṅgāsana* (cobra pose), a backbend, is the quintessential pose to help reposition the lumbar vertebrae and their associated tissues. We have seen already how the serpent power (kuṇḍalinī) is essential to personal vitality, and cobra pose serves to realign and energize the lumbar spine. We will see in the next chapter how all backbend movements help activate the adrenal glands at the top of the lumbar column; the adrenals are small but potent glands that govern levels of arousal and impact the subtle body.

In order to counter the deleterious effects of slumpasana, it is valuable to mobilize the lumbar spine and pelvis. The pelvis and sacrum move together like a swing set, given their ability to rock forward and back on the heads of the femurs. Many different types of movement express this undulation of the pelvis. For instance, one of the foundational movements in African dance involves arching the spine forward and back, initiated by a rhythmic rocking of the pelvis. The cat-cow movement in yoga, done from a hands-and-knees position, involves a similar anterior and posterior rolling of the pelvis. Sūryanamaskāra (sun salutation), the crux of all vinyāsa, is more demanding than cat-cow but nevertheless involves moving between posterior tilt (upward-facing dog pose) and anterior tilt (downward-facing dog pose). The front-back swivel of the pelvis promotes a wash of nutrient-rich fluids into the lumbosacral junction and intervertebral disks of the low back. This kind of motion is critical to maintaining fluid motion at the lumbosacral hinge and to hydraulically pumping the vital essence of life through the entire spinal column.

PRACTICE

Spinal Undulation

The following sequence brings fluid motion to the spinal base. Thomas Hanna, a student of Moshe Feldenkrais, taught pelvic tilts in a supine position with the knees bent in a movement called spinal undulation. Increasing fluid motion at the lumbosacral junction and within the stout and weighty lumbar vertebrae helps maintain the health of the intervertebral disks.

Lie on your back in śavāsana and fully relax all your muscles by letting the weight of your bones drop. Release the weight of your buttocks into the floor and sense the weight of your sacrum sinking downward. Notice the juncture of your lumbar spine and your sacrum. Do you feel compressed at L5–S1? Does your sacrum feel jammed or restricted, or does it rest comfortably on the floor?

Next, bend your knees and set your feet hip-width apart. Begin the undulation on inhalation by rocking your pelvis toward your tailbone and arching your lower back. This is anterior tilt. Breathe into your abdomen so that your belly expands as described in the "Breathing into the Abdominopelvic Balloon" exercise (see page 146). On the exhalation, scoop your pelvis into posterior tilt by rounding your lumbar spine and pressing your lower spine into the floor. Continue back and forth combining breath with movement as in all vinyāsa. In particular, observe the range of motion at your lumbosacral junction. Sense any binding, pain, or compression at the base of your spine. Imagine your pelvis to be a swing on a swing set and note the relative ease of motion as your pelvis alternates between anterior and posterior tilt.

With each exhalation concentrate on pressing the area below your navel straight back toward your spine. This strengthens and tones the deep musculature of the abdomen. Contracting the lower abdomen is essentially the "seed" movement for uḍḍīyāna bandha, to be reviewed in the following chapter. In the spinal undulation, note that with every inhalation, your lower back muscles contract as your belly rises and spreads. This movement strengthens the lower spinal muscles. Make the movement as fluid as you can. Let your breath initiate the movement rather than forcing it muscularly. Repeat this rocking movement six to ten times.

Then interlock your fingers behind your head as if you are preparing for an old-fashioned sit-up. Cradle your head in your hands and on an exhalation manually lift your head off the floor, draw your elbows toward one another, and round your entire spine. Curl your upper thoracic spine off the floor, including the third and fourth thoracic vertebrae (T3 and T4), which lie between your scapulae. On the inhalation roll your spine back down to the floor vertebra by vertebra. Then arch your lumbar spine by rocking your sacrum toward your tailbone (anterior tilt). Simultaneously arch your cervical spine as in *matsyāsana* (fish pose). Repeat this supine vinyāsa five or six times, integrating breath with movement. Keep the movements soft and rhythmic and avoid muscular force. When you are done, extend your arms and legs out in Śavāsana (corpse pose). Observe a feeling of expansion in both your sacral and cervical regions.

Untucking the Tail

The coccyx, or tailbone, articulates with the sacrum at the posterior end of the spine. While we have covered the tailbone relative to the mūlādhāra chakra in the last chapter, it is important to investigate here the effects of slumpasana on the tailbone.

The energy invested in the tail of four-legged creatures is considerable. The tail—inclusive of the sex glands, the urine-secreting ducts, and pelvic floor—is used to mark territory, attract the opposite sex, and express emotion. In humans the tailbone, while seemingly superfluous and obsolete, galvanizes and directs pulsating rhythms within the subtle body.

The coccyx shares a cartilaginous articulation with the sacrum, enabling infinitesimal motion. The coccyx, along with its adjoining structures, is highly sensitive and responsive. If you have ever slipped on ice or fell from a perch and landed on your tailbone, you know how painful blunt force is to the coccyx. In haṭha yoga, the tip of the spine is a polestar for navigating movement, especially intrinsic motion relevant to the spine and spinal fluid. In Āyurvedic healing there is a marma point, a specialized pressure point that governs the flow of prāṇa, at the lowest tip of the coccyx. This point, the *trika marma*, is used to reduce sacral pain, pelvic floor dysfunction, and lower back pain (see fig. 2.8). The dormant kuṇḍalinī can be activated by the trika marma as the coccyx curls forward into the pelvic floor, stirring the slumbering serpent.

Chronic backward tilt of the pelvis in sitting causes the tailbone to drag downward and press against the seat. This can wreak havoc on the vital structures around the pelvic floor and spinal tip. Sitting on the tailbone can numb or deaden the lower spinal nerves, and stunt pulsation that flows at the spinal base. The fine neural filaments at the posterior tip of the spine are delicate and may suffer compression over the course of long periods of sitting. Notice in figure 3.3, Model A, how the tailbone is tucked under in a posterior tilt causing compression at L5 and S1. In Model B the lumbar is shown with appropriate anterior curvature. Notice as the pelvis rocks to anterior tilt, L5 and S1 move into the body, and the coccyx suspends off the seat.

Any forward tilt of the pelvis offloads the pressure against the tip of the coccyx and allows for greater range of motion and circulation of fluids around the spinal base. By releasing compression within the ligaments and connective tissues that hold the tailbone and sacrum in place, the contents inside the pelvis—the bladder, colon, and uterus or prostate—can decompress and "float." Anterior pelvic tilt spreads the perineum, helping to reduce hypertonicity in the musculature at the base of the spine. Downward dog pose is the preeminent pose for shifting the pelvis into anterior tilt (simply called dog tilt), stretching the pelvic diaphragm and allowing the pelvic viscera to suspend.

PRACTICE

Nodding the Sacrum, Mobilizing the Tail

This series of poses serves to articulate the lumbosacral hinge and to generate extension in the lumbar spine. While helping to regain anterior lumbar curvature, this set of poses is designed to release the pelvic diaphragm and pelvic organs, and reduce constriction at L5-S1.

Adho Mukha Śvānāsana

To stretch the delicate tissues around your tailbone and mobilize your lumbosacral region, move into adho mukha śvānāsana (downward-facing dog pose). In order to broaden your pelvic floor, set your feet to the width of your mat and turn your toes slightly inward. This will help spread the connective tissues that secure the coccyx. Then rise up onto the mounds of your big toes and lift your heels and sitting bones (recall the correlation between pelvic heels and foot heels explored in the last chapter). By elevating your sitting bones, your pelvis will roll into an anterior tilt and your sacrum will pitch into the body (in anatomical nomenclature, this movement is called sacral nutation). For students who are tight in the hamstrings and low back, the lumbar spine will simply round up to the ceiling in the slumpasana shape. Those students should bend their knees, swivel their pelvis into dog tilt, and work to shift their lumbar into a concave position.

While bending your knees and rocking your pelvis into front tilt, feel the lateral spreading of your pelvic diaphragm and sense an opening inside the "cave" of your sacrum. This will allow your sacral region to become hollow and wide. Imagine you are opening a miniature parachute inside your pelvic cavity. Stay for one to two minutes.

PRACTICE

Supported Bridge Pose

In order to mobilize the juncture of L5-S1, generate extension in the low back, and help reestablish lumbar curvature, supported bridge pose is invaluable. Begin by lying on your back with your knees bent and your feet hip-width apart. Lift up into *setu bandhāsana* (bridge pose) and set a yoga block under your sacrum. If you have a history of compression in your lumbar spine, start with the block on its lowest side. For greater stability, set two blocks just lateral to your SI joints under your ilia. If you use two blocks, be sure that the blocks are under your pelvis but off of your sacrum. If you are using one block, place the block under your sacrum and posterior superior iliac spines (PSIS). Be sure that L5 is not on the block but tractions away from the sacrum. Bridge pose is an antidote to L5-S1 compression and the slumpasana. Actively press your feet to the floor and lengthen your side waist away from the block toward your head. If you have considerable tension in your lower back or contraction in your iliopsoas, the last few lumbar vertebrae will be reluctant to move and it may be painful. Should you get pain in your low back, reduce the height of the block or elevate your feet using blocks or a bolster.

If you do not experience pain, then bind your upper thighs with a strap in such a way that your legs remain hip-width apart. Set the block on its tall end and straighten your legs, firming your upper thighs against the strap. While more demanding (and you must be warmed up to do this), the straight leg variation of bridge pose will encourage greater extension of your lumbar spine and provide further traction for L5-S1. Hold the pose for one to two minutes. Remove the strap before lowering your pelvis to the floor to rest.

Apāna and the Large Intestine

In the body, all that flows downward is governed by *apāna*, a downward-moving, expulsive force. In the natural world, the descent of apāna includes rivers that flow down to the sea, mudslides, rain, avalanches, rockslides, fallen trees, and downdrafts of wind current. In the lower abdomen where apāna resides, the downward movements of birth, menstruation, defecation, and urination are subject to a similar gravitational pull.

Apāna is centered primarily in the large intestine, and regularity of elimination is critical for health in the body (fig. 3.4). The propulsive force of apāna is closely linked to the sacrum, as the terminal portion of the colon conforms to the shape of the anterior sacrum. Just in front of the coccyx and attaching to the tailbone are three cylindrical rings of the anal sphincter muscle. Thus, movement within the sacrum and tailbone couple with movement of the colon. The practice of mūla bandha helps to regulate peristaltic rhythm within the colon and strengthen its muscular walls. In movements such as spinal undulation, cat-cow, or the combination of upward dog and downward dog, the colon is pumped along with the surrounding muscular-skeletal structures.

When the large intestine is compacted, people suffer from constipation. Constipation not only impairs digestive flow, but also affects cardiovascular and respiratory rhythms. Thus, when the downward flow of apāna is blocked, the flow of prāṇa in the lungs is compromised and breathing becomes shallow and restricted.

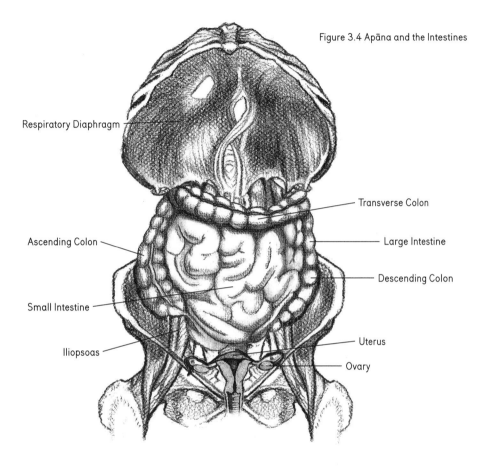

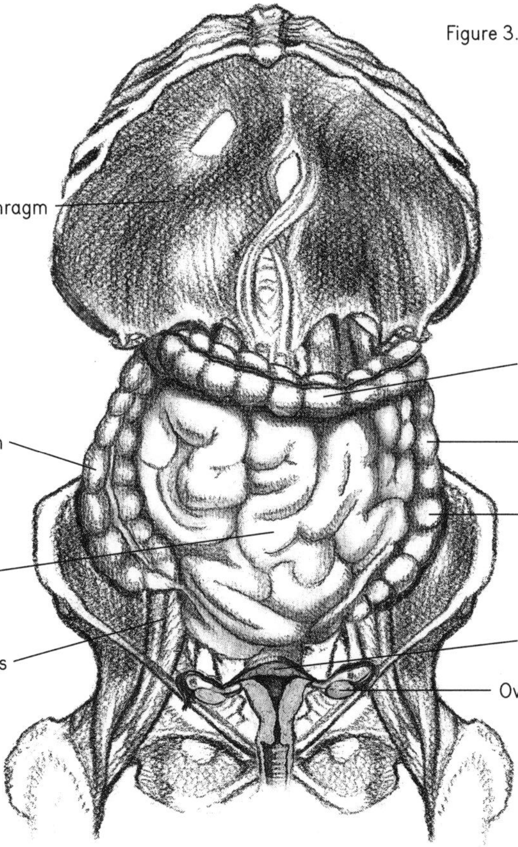

Figure 3.4 Apāna and the Intestines

The Large Intestine and the Lungs

At first glance it would seem that the lungs and large intestine are unrelated organs. Yet in the way that groundwater in lakes, rivers, and oceans determines levels of humidity in the atmosphere by way of evaporation, the "water table" of the large intestine plays a role in the circulation of bodily fluids conveyed by the lungs. In yoga and Chinese medicine, the lungs and the large intestine are homologous or paired. In the energetic system of Chinese medicine, each of the internal organs is paired, for it is thought that overall physiological function is due to a dynamic balance of yin and yang. The large intestine is yang. Hollow and hulking, the large intestine is responsible for the mechanical pumping of foodstuff toward elimination. Its contractile motion facilitates elimination at the base of the body. The lung is yin. It is blood-filled, delicate, and responsible for oxygenating the bloodstream. The lungs draw in oxygen at the top of the body. Both organs are involved in absorption and dissemination of fluid and regulation of the body's circulatory system.

In the same way that the large intestine and lungs correlate in traditional Chinese medicine, apāna in the pelvic cavity is counterpart to prāṇa in the thoracic cavity. When absorption and peristaltic movement in the colon are optimal, absorption of prāṇa in the lung tissue is enhanced.

A yoga practice should invariably begin by mobilizing the colon and releasing congestion in the lower digestive tract. To circulate prāṇa through all the nādīs, it is imperative that the bowels function regularly. During the exhalation phase of yogic breathing, as the abdomen deflates, breath is expelled from the lungs and the colon is set in motion.

In the practice of yoga, twisting poses are ideal to activate apāna, given their wringing effect on the lower abdomen. Twists help squeeze and churn the colon, encouraging a series of wavelike contractions within the intestinal folds. Twists are like mini-colonics and help to propel chyme through the colon. When there is balanced peristaltic activity in the large intestine, neither too slow nor too fast (spasmodic), proper elimination is assured. Although it is counterintuitive, upside-down positions promote the downward course of apāna. Inversions such as headstand and shoulderstand reverse the effects of gravity due to the way the triangular sacrum is turned "right side up," unmooring the structures within the pelvic cavity, loosening the bowels, and helping to relieve constipation.

Congestion in the large intestine may also result from emotional holding. Repressed emotion linked to fear, shame, grief, sadness, or condemnation interrupt the body's capacity for regular elimination.

People who are afraid to *let go*, either of their material belongings or of their feelings, are prone to obstruction in their lower gastrointestinal tract. It is all too common that bound emotions or squelched feelings burrow into the lower spine and pelvis causing both musculoskeletal and visceral knots.

The Importance of Letting Go

The idea behind letting go is part of the very foundation of the Aṣṭāṇga eight-limbed path. Nonhoarding is part of the first limb of Aṣṭāṇga Yoga, which delineates right action and proper conduct (*yama*) in the social sphere. In Sanskrit, this is referred to as *aparigraha*, which literally means "nongrasping." This attribute is meant to be an antidote to greed and possessiveness. In this country people are known to amass abundant material belongings, and most basements and attics are caches of accumulated stuff. Material possessiveness may be coupled with physiological holding and psychological clinging. For people not only collect and hoard physical belongings but withhold sentiments and innermost feelings. In the body, held-back or stuffed emotion can manifest as clogging and surplus in the lower intestinal area.

PRACTICE

Colonic Twists

These revolving poses, the first upright and the second supine, aid in mobilizing the pelvic viscera. Specifically they aim to mobilize the coils of the large intestine and to activate apānic force in the body.

Marīcyāsana III

In order to increase the movement of apāna within the large intestine, begin by sitting on the edge of a blanket with your legs straight out in daṇḍāsana (staff pose). Bend your right knee and draw it up against you in preparation for the twisting pose, *marīcyāsana III* (named for the sage Marīchi). Set your right heel as close to your sitting bone as possible, for this will serve to flex (squeeze) your ascending colon on the right side of your abdomen (see fig. 3.4). If you are tight in your hip flexors, be sure to elevate your pelvis more. Move your left leg six to ten inches to the left to create greater space for the region in your lower belly to turn. Lift and twist your torso toward your right thigh, revolving your navel toward your inner right thigh.

There are three distinct positions for entwining the left arm, listed here by increasing degree of difficulty: (1) entwine your left forearm around the outside of your right knee and shin like a coat hanger, (2) latch your left elbow to the outside of your right knee, and (3) wrap your left elbow around the outer edge of your right knee and clasp your hands together. Be sure to twist on exhalation (the apānic phase of the breath) and feel a strong wringing action below your navel. Sense and feel the way your right colon is compressed. Hold the pose for thirty seconds to a minute, then repeat on your left side. After completing both sides perform downward dog to lift and spread your abdomen.

Jaṭhara Parivartanāsana

This pose serves to revolve the lumbar spine, the abdominal organs, and endopelvic fascia. This variation involves elevating the pelvis in order to create a "hanging twist." The name *jaṭhara parivartanāsana* (revolved abdomen pose) implies revolving the coils (*jaṭa*) of the intestine.

Lie on your back and prop your pelvis six to ten inches off the floor using a bolster (or a stack of blankets). Set the bolster perpendicular to your spine with your sacrum positioned at the left side of the bolster. Bend your knees and draw them into your chest. Swing your knees to the right so that you now rest on the outer edge of your right hip. Due to the way that your pelvis is propped by the bolster, your spine will gain increased suspension and traction. In the twist, draw your knees toward your right shoulder so that the abdominopelvic rotation will be more pronounced. Keep your shoulders and upper spine on the floor and spiral your abdomen to the left, away from your knees. By elevating your pelvis and combining this elevation with rotation and traction, the connective tissues around your large intestine and bladder (and uterus in women) are mobilized and receive an ample supply of blood.

Hold the position for two minutes and then swing your knees up to center. Shift your pelvis to the far right side of the bolster before revolving your knees to the left. Afterward rest in bridge pose for several minutes with your pelvis propped in the middle of the bolster and direct your breath into your pelvic organs.

The Craniosacral Dynamic

In the subtle body, a band of light illuminates the body's interior. This light is hailed as the goddess Chitriṇī, the Radiant or Lustrous One, and is equated with pure intelligence. This innermost conduit of light surges like a tide, alternately expanding and narrowing. Anatomically, we know that the spinal cord is the neurological nucleus of the body, set plumb through the vertebral column. In the energy body, we could imagine the fluid that cushions the brain and spinal cord to be like liquid light. It emerges from the back of the brain, oozes down the spinal cord, to be pumped upward via the motion of the sacrum. This vital fluid, called the cerebrospinal fluid (CSF), is translucent and clear. CSF may have a correlation to the divine nectar (amṛta) described in ancient yoga texts that animates the subtle body.

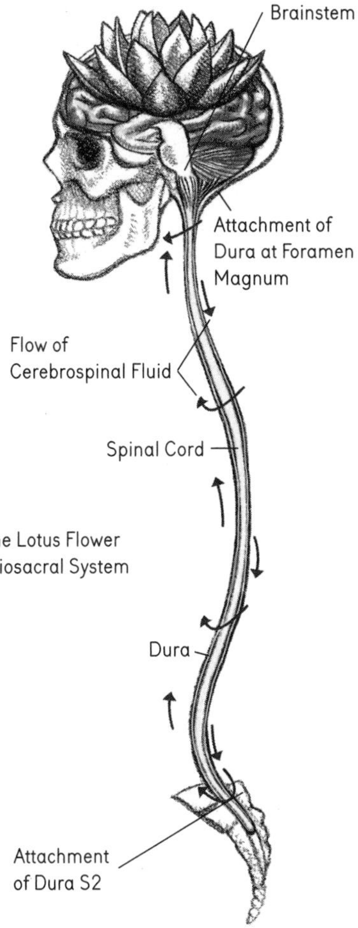

Figure 3.5 The Lotus Flower and the Craniosacral System

The analogy of the water lotus stalk and lotus blossom is comparable to the sacrum, spinal cord, and brain (fig. 3.5). Each is suspended in a fluid substratum. Similar to the way that a lotus stalk is made buoyant by the water that surrounds it, the spinal cord, within the protective caging of the vertebral column, is buoyed by CSF. The spinal fluid flows from the skull to sacrum via a reciprocal tension membrane that has its own pump, independent of the heartbeat. Motion of the CSF is partially propelled via movement within the sacrum, and thus any positions that enhance sacral motion in yoga, tai chi, and other disciplines support the rhythmic surge of this fluid.

Spinal Cord and the Lotus Bloom

In states of samādhi, yogis discovered that the most intrinsic rhythms within the body are both fluid and electric. Liquid-electric rhythms were thought to animate the subtle body since the time of the Vedas and were evoked as the deities *Soma* (water, moon) and *Agni* (fire, sun). The essential force of life, the prāṇa, was imagined to be liquid and luminous like reflected sparkles of sunlight shimmering on an inner sea of miniature waves. In Indian spirituality water has always been deemed a healing medium.

The ocean, tropical pools, and forest springs are auspicious spots for *sadhus* (holy men) and *sādhakas* (practitioners) to perform their routines—chanting mantras, performing prāṇāyāma, and invoking elemental powers. Growing naturally in the pools of the forest grove, the water flower became the metaphor for enlightenment. The aquatic flower is both exquisite and refined. Its delicate leaves and petals suspend with utmost sensitivity and grace, just as the pithy structures within the body, the brain, brain stem, and spinal cord suspend like interior pendants. The experience of samādhi, for all its buoyant effulgence, gave way to countless narratives of the chakras blooming like lotus flowers.

It is remarkable that the brain and spinal cord are afloat. They bob imperceptibly on the movement of internal vibratory waves in the way that a water lily oscillates when wind ripples across the surface of a pond. The brain and spinal cord are constantly changing shape due to the fluctuating field of the CSF and shifts in the surrounding connective tissues. Cerebral spinal fluid ebbs and flows like tides that rise and then recede along the shoreline. In fact in craniosacral therapy, the filling and emptying phases of the CSF between sacrum and skull are simply called tides. In yoga, all postural movements and breathing techniques help to support the internal tides within the spine's fluid interior.

This precious internal fluid that lubricates and suspends the spinal cord is enclosed in a membranous sheathing called the dura. The dural stocking is a semielastic tube, like the fibrous stalk of the lotus flower, that covers the brain and spinal cord. The dura anchors in two key places: to the base of the skull at the rim of the foramen magnum (where the brain stem passes through the cranial base), and to the sacrum at the second sacral segment (see fig. 3.5). William Sutherland, a pioneer in the field of craniosacral studies, called this connection between the skull and sacrum the "core link." For the ancient yogic seers, movement within the sacrum at the second chakra is closely tied—skeletally, neurologically, and spiritually—to the resplendent opening of the crown chakra.

The Craniosacral Core Link

The hula dance from Hawaii, circular movements within tai chi, and the rhythmic wavelike movements of the spine in African dance all involve the craniosacral connection. Children frequently rock themselves to sleep via rhythmic nodding motions of their head. The spinal undulation (guided on page 88) generates a gentle rocking movement between skull and sacrum. It supports relaxation and induces a parasympathetic response.

The sacrum is connected to the skull by a single highway of ligament called the anterior longitudinal ligament. (Fig. 2.5 shows the anterior longitudinal ligament spanning from the perineum to the respiratory diaphragm.) Ligaments hold bone to bone, and this ligament runs along the anterior bodies of the vertebrae as it snakes from the tailbone to the base of the skull. This ligament is complemented by the posterior longitudinal ligament, which travels along the posterior margin of the vertebral bodies. These two ligaments effectively sandwich the spherical bodies of the spine and intervertebral disks, thus providing cushion, elasticity, and spring to the spinal column. These ligaments are rivers of living tissue, resilient yet flexible, and their kinetic currents impact the body's central channel. They are part of the subtle body's core link, and via their reciprocal tension, skilled therapists and practitioners align and harmonize the craniosacral polarity.

Triangles and the Geometry of the Subtle Body

In Sanskrit, the word for the sacrum is *trikāsthi,* the "triangular bone." Anyone who knows trikonāsana (triangle pose) may recall that *trikon* means triangle. This reference helps us understand the energetic attributes of the sacrum. Visually, the sacrum appears as an inverted triangle; its apex, at the tip of the coccyx, points like a trowel toward the earth. The downward-pointing triangle serves to direct kinetic forces downward through the pelvis, legs, and feet into the earth.

The triangle is significant not only for the way it represents the sacrum. It is denoted in multiple geometrical graphs and symbols throughout India to suggest the generative force of all creation. One of these, the *Sri Yantra*, is an elaborate weave of interpenetrating triangles used to cultivate meditative awareness (fig. 3.6). Nine triangles are superimposed in a mesmerizing grid. The decorative device of the Sri Yantra maps two diametrical forces in the body, one governed by the sacrum and the other by the occiput. The downward-pointing sacrum embodies the inverted triangle while the occipital bone, at the top of the spine (also triangular in shape), describes the upward-pointing triangle (see fig. 7.2).

The Sri Yantra is suggestive of a twofold power, a dynamic play of opposites wherein seemingly contradictory forces are brought together and reconciled. Creation and dissolution, evolution and involution, Śiva and Śakti, high and low, base and crown exist in magnetic flux. In the philosophy of Samkhya Yoga from which Patañjali's Yoga Sutras and the Bhagavad Gītā derive, the upward-pointing triangles suggest the unmanifest, the absolute, or the male principle called *puruṣa*. The descending triangles (in keeping with the sacral shape) suggest manifestation, birth, and productivity, or the feminine principle called *prakṛti*.

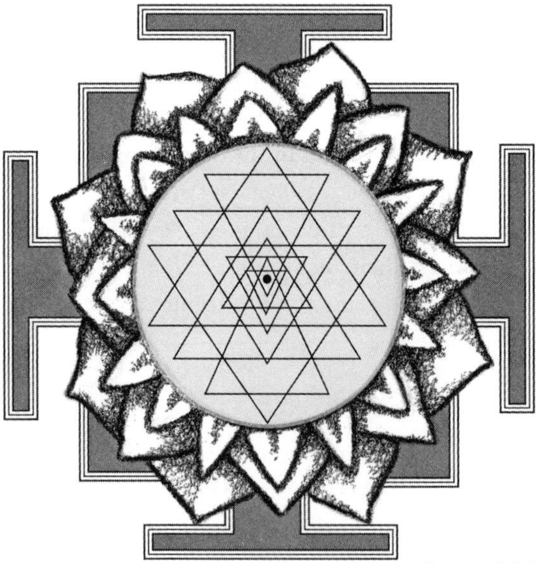

Figure 3.6 Sri Yantra and the Union of Opposites

The multiple overlapping triangles within the sacred symbol of the Sri Yantra (which translates as "auspicious form") graphically express a creative tension that is necessary to sustain all life. The yantra represents the forces at large in the overall cosmos, forces that both complement and compete. In the microcosm of the subtle body, the upward and downward triangles describe the flow of internal prānic currents. In the middle of the geometric yantra is a *bindu* (focal point or epicenter), where the two polarizing forces coincide. The yogi or meditator is meant to rest his or her *dṛṣṭi* (gaze) at this point of conjunction between ascending and descending triangular forces. In so doing the yogi abides at the still point, a singular point of harmony in the midst of opposition. The bindu is a pixel of nonduality, the dynamic center point between the manifest and unmanifest.

In the next chapter, we focus on the abdominal center and will map the abdomen as the point of convergence for all energies of the body. Like the bindu in the center of the Sri Yantra, the belly and umbilicus are equidistant between the upward rising prāṇa and the descending apāna. Its activities are centripetal and by gathering inward, it concentrates and harmonizes the primary life-force.

PRACTICE

Meditation on Inner Triangles

Assume a comfortable seated position and settle the weight of your bones on your cushion by exhaling a few times. Relax your abdomen and release any tension that might be held or stored in your diaphragm. Close your eyes and visualize an inverted triangle located within your abdomen in such a way that the apex of the triangle is the tip of your coccyx and the base of the triangle is the horizontal sheath of your respiratory diaphragm. During each exhalation, trace the path of this upside-down triangle downward to the tip of your tailbone. Initiate your breath from the span of the upper two corners of the triangle, located at the outer margin of your respiratory diaphragm.

Imagine then a second upright triangle overlaid atop this first triangle. Locate the base of this upward-pointing triangle at the level of your navel and visualize the apex located in the center of your heart. With each inhalation, feel the expansion of all three sides of this upward-pointing triangle. At the crest of the inhalation bring your awareness to the pinnacle of this upper triangle within your heart.

The lower triangle suggests *apāna vāyu,* whose downward course is charted by the out-breath, while the upward triangle conveys *prāṇa vāyu,* the "wind" of the in-breath whose abode is the heart. Last, focus your attention on the midpoint of these interlocking triangles, midway between your navel and your respiratory diaphragm. This is the bindu that relates to the fire center, or *samāna vāyu* (equalizing wind) of the solar plexus. This focal point integrates and harmonizes the ascending and descending currents in the body.

Magnify and dilate this epicenter between the opposing triangles. In time visualize your entire breath pattern initiating from this point so that it becomes the source for all the prānic currents that flow through your body. Stay for five to ten minutes.

4

THE BELLY BRAIN

The Third Chakra, the Hidden Power

The true body is the body burnt up, the spiritual body. The unity is not organic-natural unity, but the unity of fire . . . melting apparent surfaces away, and displaying the infinite which was hid.

—Norman O. Brown, *Love's Body*[1]

The abdomen is the furnace of the body, a source of scintillating energy, singled out in yoga practice as the plexus of personal power. The abdomen is the source of tapas, digestive fire and yogic fire. Underneath the hood of the diaphragm, combustion occurs via an admixture of organs and glands. Just as the flames of a fire are difficult to control, the abdominal fires are difficult to regulate. Given the pervasive influence the abdomen has on the body, tensions within the third chakra, the *maṇipūra chakra,* tend to be intractable.

The Vulnerable Belly

Throughout the evolution of biological structure, all creatures whether the triceratops or the tree frog, an alligator or an armadillo, a shark or an inchworm, never expose their bellies. For animals to expose any part of their front is to make the organism vulnerable to the risk of attack. Our pet canine and feline friends only roll over to receive a benevolent belly scratch because they are not driven by the will to survive. In the wild, pups or cubs may roll over in play, but not for long, for instinctually they know that they must orient themselves on all fours, their vitals oriented to the ground in a posture of protection. So powerful is the urge to guard the heart, lungs, and gut that a coyote or wolf, when showing deference to the alpha male (or female), will not turn over but will hunker low to the ground, flattening its body in submission.

In all vertebrates, the processes of the spine jut backward in order to fortify and protect the organs and central life-supporting blood vessels. The dorsal (back) shields the ventral (front), never the reverse. With its belly oriented toward the ground, an animal safeguards its guts—its life-sustaining third chakra—at all costs.

Homo sapiens, however, have evolved to an upright and vertical stance. While critical for the evolution of our brain, the unique and precarious bipedal posture exposes the entire front side of our body rendering us vulnerable to any oncoming frontal force, real or imagined. Segments of our ventral side have rigid bony surfaces: the pubis protects the pelvis, the sternum and ribs protect the heart and lungs, the mandible and facial bones protect the sensory organs, and the frontal bone of the skull protects the brain. However, the throat and belly are exposed, their spongy surfaces left naked and defenseless. (The throat is actually buffered by the tiny hyoid bone, but given that it is no larger than a wishbone, it doesn't provide much armor.)

These two gaps in our structural armor—the belly and the throat—spawn feelings of helplessness, both physically and mentally. In this light, the third chakra in the gut, the maṇipūra, and the fifth chakra in the throat, the *viśuddha,* are paired (see fig. 7.5). A gnawing sense of uneasiness can have a corrosive effect on both belly and throat. It is ironic that the vulnerable belly is the very source for personal power, a power that is centered in the solar plexus.

The Palace of Jewels

The name of the third chakra, *maṇipūra,* is typically translated as "the power center." This may not be a surprise, given the value that human culture places on power: monetary power, charismatic power, national power, personal power, and physical power. In the body, the abdomen is the source of command, influence, and self-will. In light of the vulnerability of the unprotected abdomen just mentioned, how could the belly be the source of such pervasive influence on both mind and body?

Figure 4.1 Kidney, Adrenal Glands, and the "Palace of Jewels"

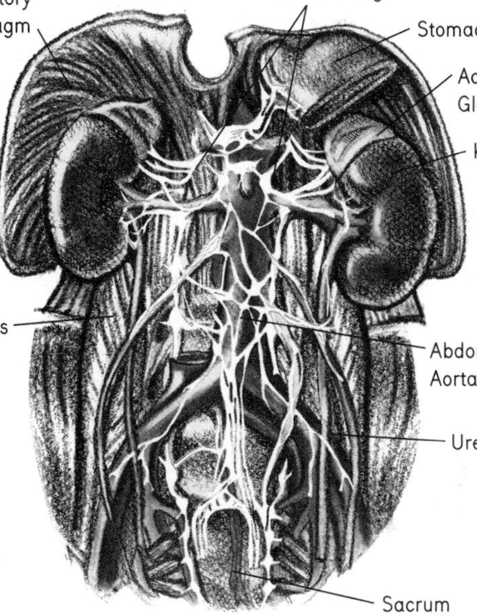

The word *maṇipūra* in Sanskrit literally translates as the "place of many riches" or "palace of jewels." In yoga practice, this reflects the view that our regal power (to be cultivated by the rigors of *rājayoga,* the "royal path of yoga") is concentrated in the solar plexus. In the back of the solar plexus are two glands, each no larger than a super ball, that have considerable sway over the body's biological rhythms. The adrenal glands, part of the hormonal system, are where instinctual impulses relating to survival get carried out. They are superconductors of biological energy, relaying high-speed signals throughout the body to take action.

Buried in the thicket of the kidney and adrenal complex is a ganglion of nerves, a neurological chain resembling a necklace of jewels (fig. 4.1). This cache of nerves drapes like a bodice set deep against the iliopsoas muscles, the abdominal aorta, and the anterior spine. It is a repository of magnificent power, ruler over the body's innermost will to live.

PRACTICE

Sensing Your Belly

This position brings a feeling of ease to the third chakra within the abdominal region. In the prone position, you will notice how your entire belly can disengage from muscular tension as you let your guard down.

Lie on your belly in śavāsana and center your head by resting your forehead on the back of one hand as you stack one hand on top of the other. Begin with your toes turned under onto the floor as in the broken-toe pose variation of vajrāsana (thunderbolt pose). Push out through your heels to lengthen the backs of your legs. Slowly then extend your feet so that the tops lay on the floor. Align the center of your forehead with the center of your pelvis. Allow the weight of your abdomen to descend into the floor. Like a parachute that has come down from the sky, notice the way your belly drops and widens. Feel the movement of your respiratory diaphragm as the weight of your lower ribs makes contact with the floor. Sense and feel every part of your chest and belly, as you breathe against the floor. Observe how your diaphragm and the organs below your diaphragm spread laterally. Then pin your pubic bone to the floor and lengthen the skin below your navel toward your chin. This spawns the movement of *uḍḍīyāna bandha*. Stay in this pose for two to five minutes, then roll onto your back without raising your head off the floor and notice the space, width, and ease that pervade your belly.

The Ram

The totem animal that symbolically resides in the third chakra is the ram. Invested with a raw, driving muscular force, the ram is the epitome of core strength. Willful, stubborn, and equipped with a capacity for relentless exertion, the ram in the abdomen represents the force of the will. Any parent who has accomplished the formidable task of rearing a child has witnessed the onset of the will at about eighteen months (into the terrible twos) and seen it flourish between the ages of four and six (sometimes lasting into the teens, twenties, and beyond!). Developmentally, as the child learns to stand firmly on his or her feet, the self-supporting posture creates feelings of autonomy. When first learning to stand and waddle around, the toddler begins to express a sense of control and self-mastery. Structurally, as the two-year-old rises to stand on both feet, the lumbar plexus, psoas, kidney, and adrenal region engage in order to coordinate the upright stance without falling. As the child learns to walk across the floor, powerful kinesthetic urges relating to self-governance in the third chakra are made manifest.

Concurrent with these physiological and structural changes, the egoic self (*ahaṅkāra*) undergoes an elaborate and complex process of construction. The word *aham* refers to "I," and *kara* means "to do." Selfhood, or the "self-doer," arises in part from impulse-driven, initiating centers in the body located below the diaphragm.

Because the forces entrusted in the will have such extensive ramifications (no pun intended), impacting thought, emotion, and behavior, the dynamics of the third chakra are difficult to navigate. The stubborn, unrelenting nature of the ram is nearly inexhaustible. The drive of the human will is equally tenacious, and the force and determination it shows are astounding. Thus, in Patañjali's yoga, the last of the five afflictions (*kleśas*) that inhibit a yogi from full illumination is attachment to life (*abhiniveśa*). Yoga practice involves mindful consideration of the urges, fears, and goals of this self-doer.

Like male rams competing for dominance and rights to a herd of gorgeous ewes, much of the motivating force within the third chakra is libidinal. To a great extent, the adrenal glands in the upper abdomen oversee the production of sex hormones in both men and women. In terms of sexual function, the lower two chakras are the implementers of the libidinal drive, whereas the third chakra is the biochemical brain that governs sexual behavior.

The Adrenal Brain

The adrenal glands perch like little yellow ski hats atop the kidneys, add-ons to the renal organs (see fig. 4.1). Part of the intricate complexity of the endocrine system that functions via a hierarchy of signals and countersignals, the adrenal glands play a significant role in self-regulation. Like battery packs, they flank the spine at the level of the dorsal lumbar curve, where the twelfth thoracic vertebra and first lumbar vertebra intersect (see fig. 5.2). This is where the spine has its greatest capacity for spring and propulsion. If you have ever experienced real fear, then you can surely recall the feeling of constriction in your upper solar plexus, just below your respiratory diaphragm. Any experience of fear activated by the adrenal glands can cause this area to clench, for the body's innate response to threat is to protect its vital organs, including the soft-bodied abdominal viscera. Anxiety and fear trigger the jitters. Patañjali in his treatise on yoga, The Yoga Sutras, identified this agitation as *citta vṛtti,* or fluctuations in the mind. Yet feelings of distress in the solar plexus underlie mental anxiety. Pertaining to abdominal jitters, we have the descriptive analogy of "getting butterflies," yet this comparison is misleading, for it is far too pleasant a reference. The experience is more like getting the mosquitoes, for the sensation is nervy, grating, and irritable—the awful anticipation of getting stung or attacked by something you cannot quite see. Under stressful circumstances, a gnawing malaise can infect the adrenal plateau of the solar plexus. Thus, the jewel-like attribute of the maṇipūra chakra loses its luster and becomes tarnished by worry and despair.

The Adrenals and the Spiritual Warrior

Composed more than twenty-five hundred years ago, the story of Arjuna at battle in the Bhagavad Gītā relates the physiology of traumatic stress. In the anticipatory moments prior to battle when Arjuna looks over the battle demarcation line and sees his kinsmen on the other side—fathers, grandfathers, uncles, sons, brothers, and his guru—he experiences paralyzing fear in his solar plexus. He tells his spiritual counselor, Kṛṣṇa, "My legs give way, my mouth dehydrates, my body trembles and shakes, my hair bristles . . . my skin becomes hot and irritated, my mind scatters, and I can no longer stand."[2] This passage describes the constriction phase of the traumatic response. Overwhelmed by fear, Arjuna's nerve endings, his breathing, circulation, and posture are plagued by tension. A surge of biochemical secretions from the adrenal complex prompts him to lose touch with himself, an experience common in the dissociating stage of trauma, which is why he at last proclaims, "I am unable to remain as I am."

The adrenals are the brain of the lower three chakras, whose intelligence is calibrated to reproduce, defend, and ensure survival. The glandular secretions of the adrenals accelerate the sympathetic nervous system, a branch of the autonomic nervous system along the thoracic and lumbar spine that governs states of arousal. In the fight-or-flight response the adrenals secrete epinephrine and norepinephrine (along with steroids), which increase heart rate, elevate blood pressure, and increase breathing.

For centuries, one of the primary objectives of a yogi has been to disrupt and redirect the physiological potency of the adrenal pulse that imparts such dramatic changes on the nervous, cardiovascular, digestive, and immune systems. In traditional yoga practices, numerous disciplines and techniques are used to monitor, arrest, or snuff out the biological spark that initiates from the third chakra. If the yogi does not regulate the adrenal charge through both physical and psychological means and direct it toward altruistic and spiritual activities, then he or she is at the whim of instinctual and impulsive drives. Like Arjuna confronted with battle, gut-level responses in the body can be ungovernable, overwhelming, or paralyzing.

In yoga training, the foremost means to mollify the might of the adrenal surge is to not commit harm, either to oneself or to others. The complex ambivalence that Arjuna grapples with on the battlefield is due to his moral imperative not to harm. Yet groomed by the warrior caste he was born into, his duty is to fight. Nonviolence (*ahiṃsā*) is the first of the yamas, the moral ethics given at the outset of the eight-limbed path of Aṣṭāṅga Yoga enumerated by Patañjali.

Abstaining from sexual activity, practicing vegetarianism, chanting the name of God 108 times, retaining the breath, retracting sensory awareness, and performing rigorous āsana are all ways to curb the flames of the adrenal fires. Along with physical tapas, mindful regulation of thought, action, and behavior helps check levels of arousal leading to states of anger, aggression, animosity, competitiveness, and so on.

Another way to tame the adrenals is through the use of intoxicants. In northern India, Śiva cults smoke copious amounts of ganja in ritual worship. The combination of *bhakti* yoga (the yoga of devotion) and cannabis consumption serves to quell levels of adrenal activation and mitigate feelings of sexual desire.

Gandhi's Tapas

Mahatma Gandhi championed nonviolence in his campaign of *satyāgraha*, his "commitment to truth," countering British rule in the 1940s. It is interesting to note that Gandhi's greatest tapas was fasting. During the march toward freedom, Gandhi's hunger strikes totaled seventeen. Hunger, and its correlate taste, is a most basic human desire. In order to counter the pull of desire, traditional yogis follow an inner promise (*vrata*) that involves devotion, nonharming, fasting, and the restraint (yama) of conduct and thought. Fasting is a powerful way to sublimate the surge of adrenaline as it shuts down the body's process of synthesizing food and thereby alters physical and mental energy. "There can be no room for selfishness, anger, lack of faith, or impatience in a pure fast," Gandhi once wrote.[3]

As part of a discipline of personal austerity, fasting (including reducing or limiting one's diet) is thought to transform the physical tissues of the body, the psyche and spirit. In the Bhagavad Gītā the discipline of tapas and abstinence of food lead to insight (*prajñā*). "Sensuous objects fade, when the subtle body refrains from food, taste lingers, but it too fades, for the one who has witnessed the supreme, the totality, the all-inclusive."[4]

PRACTICE

Solar Plexus Breathing

Monitoring the tick of adrenal rhythm is paramount to altering the internal body clock. The very first stage in working with the potency of the adrenals involves developing sensitivity for the dominion and sway of the solar plexus beneath the diaphragm. This exercise guides you to sense the quality of presence within your solar plexus, the lair of the adrenal glands.

Assume a comfortable seated position so that you have ample support for your pelvis and lower spine. If you have knee strain or your lumbar spine collapses, sit in a chair or sit on the floor against a bolster propped on its end and leaning against the wall. Align the middle band of your trunk so it is not pushing forward or slumping back. Relax your jaw, throat, and tongue. Sense the space just below your diaphragm at the top of your solar plexus. Bring your fingers to the spot just below the base of your sternum in order to palpate the top of your solar plexus. This is the location of your respiratory diaphragm. As you lower your hands down, notice the atmospheric tension of your upper solar plexus. Does it feel tight, like a walnut in its shell? Does it feel quivery, twisted, loose, or vacant? Does it feel like you are on guard in this area? Relax as much as possible just below your diaphragm. Imagine your breath is a spray of mist diffuse through your belly. Aim to guide your breath to the posterior wall of your abdomen, home to the kidney and adrenal complex. Notice if a clenched, quivery, or frozen feeling persists and if the muscular tension in your upper abdomen never fully dissolves. Sit for ten minutes and afterward lie on your back in viparīta karaṇī with your legs up the wall for several minutes.

Fire and Fluidity

The kidneys, which are each approximately the size of your closed fist, are sheltered underneath the floating ribs at the back of the abdominal cavity. The kidneys are immediately below the respiratory diaphragm and against the iliopsoas muscles (see fig. 4.1). Their position in midtrunk suggests their central role in governing the body's overall level of physical energy.

While the adrenal glands oversee the body's capacity for sudden and immediate response in spurts of energy, the kidneys are the storehouse for vitality, longevity, and endurance. In light of the subtle body and the elements, it is remarkable that the adrenals and the kidneys are paired, for the adrenals are like spark plugs and are related to fire, while the kidneys are blood filters related to water. The body is perpetually seeking to regulate the effects of fire and fluidity. This requires reconciling states of exertion needing the production of heat with states of rest implying the coolness of water. This delicate balance has far-reaching effects on the body, impacting cycles of sympathetic and parasympathetic activity, blood pressure, and sleep cycles.

Within the yoga tradition, the mixture of fire and water holds an alchemical charge, one that spawns the basis of all life. There are references to the conjunction of these two elements as far back as the *Rig Veda* (1500 to 1200 B.C.E.). In some of the earliest hymns of the Vedas, fire (*agni*) is personified as the deity who has the capacity to purify and transform. Agni is ritual fire, the recipient of sacrifice; through its powers of combustion it alters any substance it touches. The Sanskrit word *agni* is similar to the English word *ignite*, and the power of ignition is suggestive of the adrenal spark plugs. (Interestingly, Agni was also the name bestowed upon India's first long-range missile capable of transporting nuclear power.)

However, the waters (*soma*) associated with the kidneys are celebrated for their capacity to heal, nourish, and illuminate. Just as agni is heat and correlates with the sun, soma is cool and inspired by the moon. Soma nourishes and provides longevity in the way that the kidneys fortify and sustain the subtle body. By filtering, regulating, and storing blood, the kidneys are reservoirs for the chi or prāṇa in the body. Like the kidney and adrenal glands, agni and soma are not contradictory or opposing forces but are concordant. Together they yield the very essence of life.

Kidney Chi

The kidneys are unique topographically because they assume the inmost deep-seated position of all organs in the body. Their location is more interior than the brain or the heart. Sequestered at the back of the abdominal cavity (behind the peritoneum) and shielded by the strong musculature of the back, the kidneys are like reservoirs that store the life-sustaining drinking water for a city. The fact that they are so deeply recessed and protected speaks to their role as storehouse of the essential fluid in the body, the life-sustaining *jing.*

In traditional Chinese medicine, the kidney and adrenal matrix govern both the body's active (yang) force and its replenishing (yin). In TCM, the kidneys are the transformers of the body. They govern reproductive function, growth, and development while assisting in the production of blood by building marrow. Physiologically the kidneys contain and filter the blood and in traditional Chinese medicine they are an integral part of the body's overall fire energy.

Traditional Chinese medicine asserts that the kidneys store the prenatal chi, the fundamental constitutional makeup we inherit from our parents that is expressed over the course of a lifetime. We could think of the kidneys as blueprints for our life-force, and since the kidney essence is limited and subject to depletion, practices such as qigong and yoga help preserve and sustain the kidney chi.

In qigong and yoga practice, vitality is first drawn upward through the feet by activating the arches and making the sole of the foot pliable. In traditional Chinese medicine, the kidney meridian, called the Bubbler or Spring of Life, travels from the Kidney 1 point on the sole of the foot along the sacred channel of the inner ankle, knee, and thigh before transiting to the organ (see figs. 1.2 and 4.2).

The Kidney and Adrenal Fatigue

If there is physical and mental depletion and the kidneys become exhausted, one is prone to infirmity and disease. Adrenal burnout and chronic fatigue are prevalent in our society: the demands of a career, mortgage, money, family, projects, and travel all take from the kidney essence. In America we are the consumer society, and this includes "consuming" the vitality of the kidneys. Stress and depletion of the kidney essence compromise neuroimmunity, digestion, sleep patterns, lymph drainage, muscle tone, and concentration levels. In a society of workaholics, it is critical to monitor fatigue levels and to spend time regularly nourishing and rebuilding the kidney chi.

Any kind of exercise regimen is valuable for promoting circulation through the kidneys, but yoga poses target the kidneys in unique and specific ways. Generally, a regular yoga practice aids in keeping the lumbar region pliable and hydrated. For instance, sūryanamaskāra (sun salutation) alternately flexes and extends the myofascia that surround the kidneys. Revolved poses such as marīcyāsana III and *ardha matsyendrāsana* (lord of the fishes pose) help to maintain proper circulation of blood and lymph in and around the kidneys. Structurally, the kidneys impact respiratory rhythm, as the kidneys directly attach to the subsurface of the diaphragm by a membranous sheathing (fig. 4.1). Should the kidneys and surrounding fascia become constricted, movement of the diaphragm during inhalations may be inhibited. A vinyāsa yoga sequence that imparts a pumping effect on the lumbar spine (via spinal undulations or cat-cow movement, for example) helps irrigate blood through the kidneys. ◈

PRACTICE

Regulating the Kidney Meridian

This pose tones and stretches the kidney meridian that travels from the sole of the foot, along the inner leg, and into the kidneys. You will need a strap and a block or bolster for this setup.

Begin by lying on your back with your knees bent and your feet flat on the floor under your knees. Loop the strap over your right heel and extend your right leg upward into *supta pādānguṣṭāsana* (reclining big toe pose). Allow your lower back and kidney region to drop into the floor and widen. Take several breaths into your midback to help irrigate blood into the kidney complex. Then straighten your left leg and stretch it along the floor. On an exhalation, sweep your right leg to the right so that your outer leg is propped on the block or bolster set under your right thigh (fig. 4.2). By moving the leg to the side you actively stretch the kidney meridian.

Inhale deeply in order to irrigate your breath into your back ribs and lower spine. Drive the inner edge of your right heel away from you to elongate the inner seam of your right leg. At the same time, flex your right foot, thereby activating the Kidney 1 point and pada bandha in the center of your plantar region. As you lengthen your inside leg,

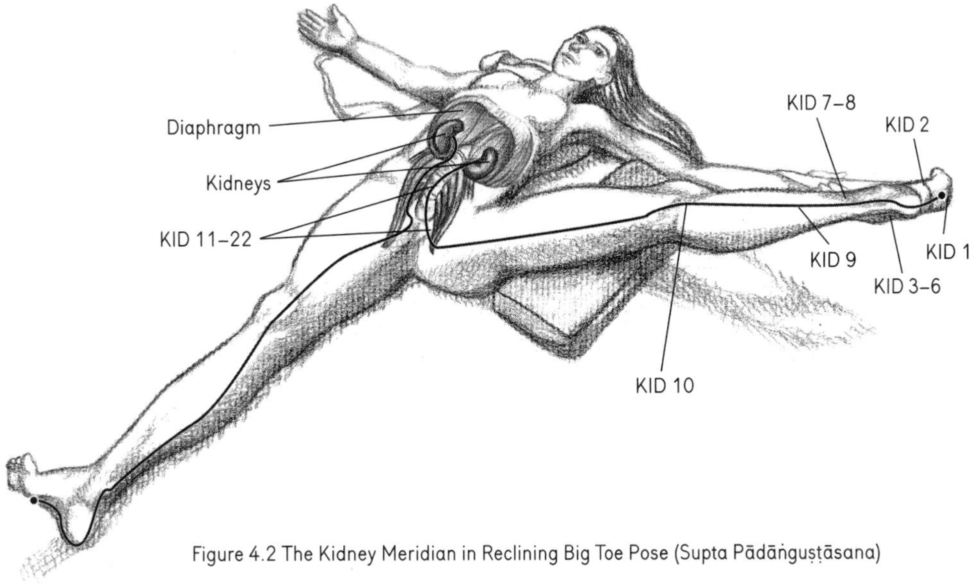

Figure 4.2 The Kidney Meridian in Reclining Big Toe Pose (Supta Pādāṅguṣṭāsana)

turn your belly to the left, away from your right leg. Feel width and space in your abdomen. Hold the pose for one to three minutes. Draw your leg back upright before switching to your other side. Repeat the pose with your left leg and then lay in śavāsana to rest.

The Iliopsoas Muscles: Flying Buttresses

Most anatomists and movement specialists agree that the iliopsoas muscles are the most intrinsic muscles in the body. They are intermediaries between legs and trunk and provide pivotal, core support. Today the word *core* has become the trademark tag for body conditioning of all kinds. Everyone is after the core. The iliopsoas muscles provide core support not only due to their central location in the body but also due to their critical role in our upright bipedal posture. Without the vertical extension of the iliopsoas muscles and the lumbar vertebrae to which they adhere, we might still be low to the ground sniffing around in search of an evening meal, our hindquarters partially coiled in preparation for fight or flight.

The support that the iliopsoas muscles provide for the lumbar spine is akin to the architectural support of the flying buttresses that flank the Notre-Dame Cathedral in Paris. In the design of the cathedral, numerous architectural struts pass from the ground to the hull of the cathedral to prop up the nave and choir. The iliopsoas muscle provides a similar support in the body, as they prop up the spine and torso from the "ground" of the legs.

The strongest hip flexor in the body, the iliopsoas begins in the inside leg, spans the hip, and fastens to the framework of the lumbar spine. One of the key myofascial connections in the body, the uppermost fibers of psoas major interweave with the fibers of the respiratory diaphragm (see fig. 2.5). This has real importance for breathing, for if the psoas muscles are taut, free motion of the diaphragm may be impaired. When the psoas muscles are lengthened, especially in backbends that involve spinal extension, the fibers of the diaphragm are stretched and one can breathe more deeply.

A fascial sleeve runs continuously from the pelvic floor along the front of the lumbar spine and up to the diaphragm. This sleeve involves the perineum, the anterior longitudinal ligament, and the deep fibers of the psoas muscle. This is valuable to keep in mind in light of the actions of mūla and uḍḍīyāna bandhas. It suggests that these two bandhas and the pelvic and respiratory diaphragms have myofascial continuity.

Thus, the Magnificent Bandha, called *mahā bandha* in the *Haṭha Yoga Pradīpikā,* involves the simultaneous lift of the pelvic floor (mūla bandha) and the iliopsoas muscle (uḍḍīyāna bandha); a downward seal of the throat (*jālandhara bandha*) is the third component.

During prāṇāyāma, and in particular when activating uḍḍīyāna bandha, the psoas is inevitably involved. Uḍḍīyāna bandha is often misunderstood as a simple contraction. By perceiving the updraft of the iliopsoas as a contraction, practitioners mistakenly tighten their gut. But uḍḍīyāna bandha involves the length and width of the entire iliolumbar region. This became clear to me in my study of Iyengar Yoga some time ago. B. K. S. Iyengar made the point that the essential movement of uḍḍīyāna bandha is accomplished in ūrdhva dhanurāsana (upward bow pose). In this backbend, the iliopsoas muscles and anterior lumbar spine are not contracted but fully lengthened. Iyengar's point was that the length of the abdominal spine and adjoining iliopsoas is instrumental to the performance of uḍḍīyāna bandha.

Freeing the Bird of Prāṇa

Falconry—common throughout Europe, Persia, and India in medieval history—became a central metaphor in yoga for how to "tame" prāṇa. The prāṇa that roams inside the body is likened to wind (*prāṇa vāyu*), and the aim of both falconery and haṭha yoga is to tether the winds of prāṇa. When the prāṇa is yoked, it serves the higher purpose of yoga, the liberation of the human spirit. In the way that a raptor in the first few launches would be unruly, uncooperative, and hard to keep still, so the prāṇa at the outset of yoga training is flighty. Via prāṇāyāma, āsana, and meditation, prāṇa is harnessed and flown in the same way that a kestrel or peregrine falcon is handled and trained.

Like the trained falcon, the wind of the breath is made to soar, hover, drop down, or be still. In the art of falconry, once a bird of prey is trained, it can fly far and wide in the sky and yet return to its perch. In the same way, a yogi, having mastered prāṇāyāma and the ability to return to the root support (via mūlā bandha), can extend his or her breath into new and far-reaching dimensions.

In the practice of āsana and prāṇāyāma, the bird of prāṇa is fettered in two vital ways. Located in the lower spinal region, these fetters (bandhas) are engaged in order to leash (and eventually unleash) the power of the prāṇa. As we saw in chapter 2, mūla bandha involves harnessing the pelvic diaphragm. Uḍḍīyāna bandha, a movement that is contiguous with the perineal lift, involves an upward suspension of the anterior lumbar spine (see fig. 4.3).

"Lock" is a poor translation of bandha, yet unfortunately it is still used in most yoga circles today. The word *bandha* (etymologically related to the English word *bind*) suggests the act of capturing, tethering, tying, or harnessing. It implies a catch that must ultimately include release. The act of bandha involves its correlate, *abandha*, which means to unfasten or liberate. Physiologically the aim of the bandhas is to open and release the breathing mechanism and to promote proper metabolic flow through the adjoining organs, glands, and vessels.

The practice of falconry would have been contemporary with the compilation of the *Haṭha Yoga Pradīpikā*, one of the most comprehensive texts on yogic techniques compiled sometime in the fifteenth century. In fact the *Pradīpikā* employs the falconry metaphor to illustrate the elusive movement of uḍḍīyāna bandha: "Uḍḍīyāna bandha is so named because by its practice the great bird of prāṇa flies upward effortlessly inside the hollow center of the suṣumnā nāḍī."[5]

Mention of the bird of prāṇa appears in other sources that predate the *Haṭha Yoga Pradīpikā*. In the Upaniṣads, which precede the *Haṭha Yoga Pradīpikā* by nearly two thousand years, there is a beautiful passage that likens the mind to a restless bird:

> Just as a bird tied by a string, after flying in various directions without finding a resting place elsewhere, settles down (at last) at the place where it is bound, so also the mind, my dear, after flying in various directions without finding a resting place settles down on the prāṇa, for the mind, my dear, is bound by the breath (*prāṇa-bandhanam*).[6]

This is one of the earliest passages suggesting that the mind (*citta*) and prāṇa are bound together.

The Flying Bandha

Uḍḍīyāna bandha is called the "flying bandha" due to the way the umbilicus area swoops backward against the spine and upward toward the respiratory diaphragm. If we think of a hovering hawk suspended over a meadow spying its lunch, a mole far in the grass below, the bird must have tremendous internal suspension to hang in midair. This suspension is accomplished not only by the span of its wings but by the muscles that comprise its abdomen and tail. In the human body the core muscles of the iliopsoas provide a similar support.

The impulse to lift upward, reversing the pull that gravity has on matter, has inspired yogis for millennia, epitomized by the stereotypical image of a yogi levitating off the ground. Many yoga poses are named for animals—cobra, frog, locust, and eagle, to name a few—as yogis imagined ways that the human body could imitate the buoyancy and ethereality of wild animals.

Uḍḍīyāna bandha is exemplified not only by a hovering hawk but by other animals that exhibit the power of upward surge. The spy-hop of a whale suggests the power of uḍḍīyāna bandha. Spy-hopping is the vertical thrust of a whale's body out of water, executed when it wants to scan the horizon. The propulsive force of a forty-five-ton animal moving vertically upward is truly awe-inspiring. The power for such a movement, against the force of gravity, requires tremendous strength in its hindquarters and tail.

To understand the force of uḍḍīyāna bandha, it is helpful to imagine other upward-surging forces of nature. The whirlwind vortex of a tornado and the updraft of air in a chimney flue suggest the power of rising prāṇa. In the abdomen, the rush of uḍḍīyāna bandha causes the organs, nerves, blood vessels, and glands to be pulled upward toward the underside of the diaphragm.

In a practical sense, why might it be valuable to perform this kind of movement? Within our sedentary culture, applying a mechanical force that will counter the downward drag of the body's interior is a good idea. All bodies are prone to collapse as they age, because gravity causes the structures of the body to slide downward toward the pelvic floor. In the abdomen, this drag can mean drooping intestines, prolapsed kidneys, and compression of the lumbar spine. David Byrne of the Talking Heads once sang, "gravity gets you down," and this is certainly true of the structures in the belly.

The pull of uḍḍīyāna bāndha is a direct means to hoist the abdominal organs and vault them upward away from the pelvic floor (fig. 4.3).

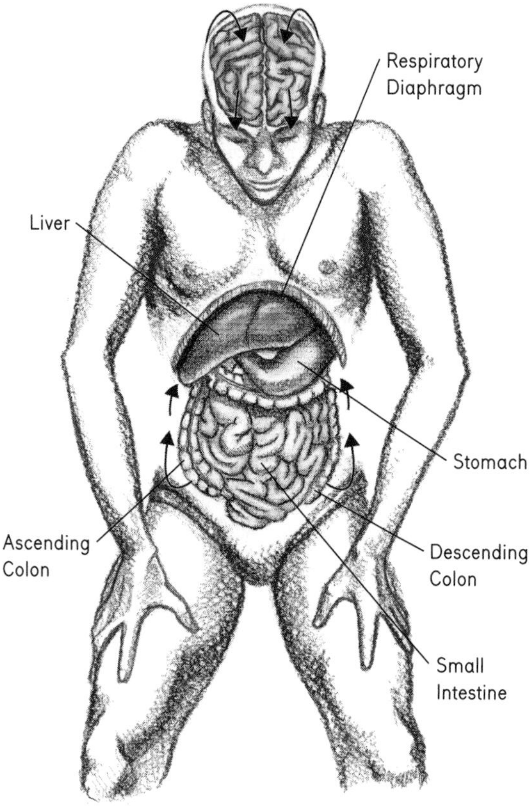

Figure 4.3 Belly Brain and Cranial Brain in Uḍḍīyāna Bandha

Yoga poses, including inversions such as headstand and shoulderstand, provide a similar antigravitational repositioning of the viscera and surrounding tissues. When we invert, the pressure gradients within the vessels, organs, and connective tissues reverse. Inversions facilitate the effects of the bandhas in a spontaneous way, imparting physiological benefits to the internal organs.

In my classes, headstand and shoulderstand are prerequisites for learning uḍḍīyāna bandha. Backbends are prerequisite due to the way they help achieve length within the iliopsoas muscles.

PRACTICE

Preparing for Uḍḍīyāna Bandha

This practice works best first thing in the morning when your stomach and intestinal tract are empty. Avoid this practice if you have high blood pressure, are menstruating or pregnant, or are prone to panic attacks.

Stand with your feet several inches wider than hip-width apart and ground the center of your heels to the floor. Activate your toes, plantar fascia, and arches as described in chapter 1. Draw in a full inhalation; with the exhalation, bend your knees and place your hands on top of your lower thighs just above your knees (see fig. 4.3). Lean your trunk forward and at the same time elongate your side waist. Set your hands so your thumbs point toward your inner thighs. Straighten your arms so that your shoulders hike up toward your ears (a shoulder position I like to call "vulture āsana").

Draw your chin down toward your breastbone while keeping the structures of your throat soft. Exhale as you push your hands solidly against your lower thighs and actively elongate your lower spine, side waist, and iliopsoas muscles. Lengthen your sacrum and tailbone toward the floor to create a hollow shape just below your navel. With each exhalation, push your hands against your thighs, press your feet to the floor, and lift your entire abdomen toward your diaphragm. In particular, the movement is accomplished at the end of each exhalation, but be careful not to strain. It is important to keep your head down at all times and your chin held to your chest (jālandhara bandha). Feel all of your abdominal organs draw back toward your spine and upward like the movement of a sheet in the wind. Hold the position for several minutes. Afterward rest in child's pose.

Scoliotic Curvature

For ideal efficiency and balance, both psoas muscles should be equal in length and strength. Because the iliopsoas attaches to the transverse processes of the lumbar vertebrae, unilateral psoas strain will often contribute to scoliosis. Almost all adults have some degree of spinal twist or spinal aberration. It would be a rare individual indeed who has lived an active life for thirty or more years and has not suffered any kind of incongruity in his or her iliopsoas and lumbar spine.

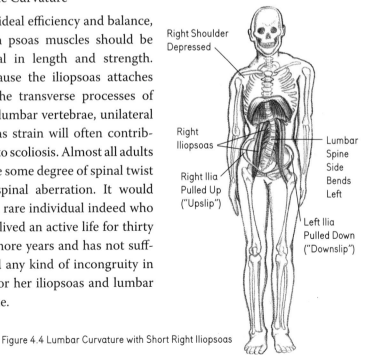

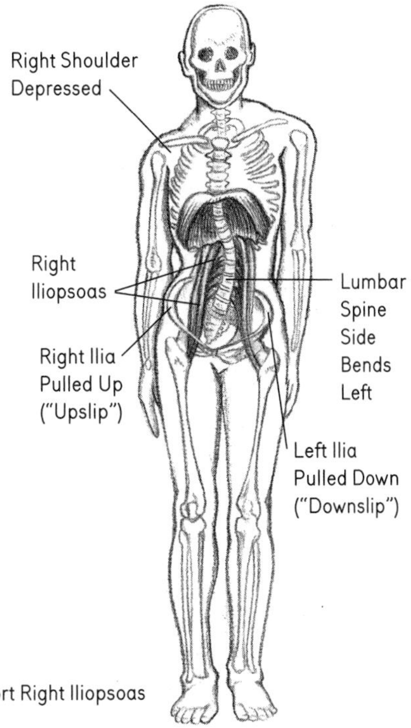

Figure 4.4 Lumbar Curvature with Short Right Iliopsoas

In the language of yoga, we could say that the right and left iliopsoas are not typically in *samasthiti,* meaning the tension in one iliopsoas muscle is typically greater than the other. One psoas may be shorter, rotated, torqued, twisted, or riddled with adhesions (fig. 4.4).

The Psoas in Three Dimensions

I recall a unique outing to the cadaver lab several years back with my colleague Richard Freeman. What could be more engaging for a pair of yogis, keen on the intricacies of the interior body, than a field trip to do dissection? It was a joy to examine with Richard, sharing insights into the labyrinth of physical structure. When observing the iliopsoas, I was struck by how ropy and spindle-like it can be. When you see the muscle drawn two-dimensionally, it looks flat, whereas in the body (in particular, in those with athletic builds), it is like thick, cyclindrical cable. I detected asymmetries (scoliotic curvature) between the right and left sides of the lumbar spine in almost all of the cadavers; the stout and ropy psoas muscle was markedly more prominent on one side.

Asymmetrical patterns in the psoas may be due to a history of trauma such as a leg break, a blow to the trunk or pelvis, or a seemingly remote and irrelevant injury such as an ankle sprain or foot injury. Frequently, lopsided psoas occurs as the result of leg dominance. In the way that people are dominant with one hand, people typically rely predominantly on one leg for support, stability, and power. Repetitive strain can cause unilateral tension in the psoas—playing soccer and kicking primarily with one leg, serving tennis balls from one side, swinging a golf club from one side, carrying children repeatedly on one hip, and so on. The psoas may also displace as a result of chronic shoulder imbalances and disparity in the middle or upper back. In short, the iliopsoas is susceptible to torsion of all kinds, and unilateral strain in the psoas will impact the position of the shoulder girdle and skull.

Most scoliotic curvature in the lumbar spine involves a left-side bend of the lower spine—that is, the right iliopsoas shortens causing the lumbar to curve to the left (see fig. 4.4). Most manuals of spinal mechanics that illustrate curvature of the spine show the lumbar spine bending to the left. The predominance of left-lumbar curvature is typically due to right-handedness. Right-side dominance may be coupled with right shoulder compression, adhesions in the right lung, compression in the right kidney, and tightness of the right iliopsoas muscle.

Fire and the Right Side of the Body

In esoteric yoga anatomy, the right side of the body is the solar side, whereas the left side is the lunar channel. The *sūrya* nāḍī (also called the *piṅgalā*) governs the right side. This is the fire channel that incorporates the logic-making left brain (as the left brain commands the right side of the body), right-handedness, and the multitasking liver. The right side generates heat through labor. Given that we are a high-octane society, a culture bent on work and production, the right border of the spine and the adjoining organs and musculature are prone to shrinkage and contraction. Specific practices in yoga and qigong aim to repair right-side stenosis. For instance, the prāṇāyāma breath called *sūrya bhedana* (literally "the solar division") involves isolating the flow of breath through the right nostril. This breath is meant to nourish and replenish the sūrya nāḍī. Another way to nourish a depleted right side, during meditation, is to envelop the entire right side of the torso in prāṇa, from the right clavicle down to the right waist.

PRACTICE

Assessing Spinal Curvature

This exercise helps to assess movement within the psoas and to determine which side of the spine may be more constricted. Insight as to which side of your spine is more restricted will give you greater somatic awareness throughout your yoga practice. Once you detect your spinal foreshortening, you can proceed carefully but diligently to generate length on your shorter side.

Lie on your back with your arms by your sides and your legs stretched out. Take several minutes to allow the weight of your bones to drop into the floor and your joints to release. Before moving, scan down the right side of your spine from your neck to your pelvis, then do the same on your left side. Can you detect any pull or shortening along one side?

Without lifting your leg, push out through your right heel, and slide the right side of your pelvis down and away from your spine as you did in the "Moving from Your Pelvic Heels" exercise in chapter 2. Slowly repeat this movement on the left side and continue by alternating legs six or seven times. Notice how the exercise resembles the motion in walking. Observe the sidebend movement of your lumbar spine and sense whether you have greater restriction on one side. The restricted side is typically the side of the shorter psoas.

Now raise your arms alongside your ears so that they are bent and in a goalpost position on the floor. Then, as you slide your right leg away from your hip along the floor, simultaneously slide your right arm along the floor over your head. Be sure to do the movement on inhalation. As you do this, notice how your lumbar and midspine sidebend to the left, in the opposite direction. Repeat on the left side. Continue slowly alternating side to side six to seven times and note how your spinal movements resemble those of a crawling lizard. Sense and feel the length of your psoas and compare your two sides. You may be able to detect that one psoas is more elastic than the other. Notice if one side of your spine presents more of a barrier to movement than your other side. This may indicate the presence of spinal curvature.

Gut Distress and the Emotions

As we have seen, the three lower chakras relate to innate biological drives critical for survival. Additionally, in the face of emotional upheaval, the powerful effects of the fight-or-flight response trigger cascading neurological impulses along the spine. A sense of malaise in the gut involves the long, wandering vagus nerve (Cranial Nerve 10). Part of the autonomic nervous system, this nerve is by far the most wide-ranging cranial nerve, as it enervates most of the organs in the body. In order to reduce levels of stress, the parasympathetic arm of the vagus nerve keeps the artillery of the sympathetic nerves, which are always loaded for response, in check. When the parasympathetic nervous system is overwhelmed, trapped emotions such as grief, fear, and helplessness adversely affect the organs. The organs are soft bodied and covered only by thin membranes. While strain can cause the outer musculature and connective tissues to shorten, as we have seen, the viscera within the body are uniquely vulnerable to emotive holding.

When the body is under threat, constriction may lodge in the stomach, liver, kidney, and intestines. When this happens, the inherent wavelike motion of the viscera, called motility, is disturbed. Functionally speaking, the organs in the gut (as well as the heart, lungs, and brain) have porous, highly absorptive interiors. This absorptive capacity leaves the organs vulnerable in the face of threat. This is especially true for children who are not yet able to process cognitively what is happening and readily internalize stress and strain. When there is emotional trauma, the organs are prone to dysfunction of various kinds: numbness, freezing, or spasmodic rigidity can result in states of irritability, spaciness, fear, restlessness, and so forth. In the face of trauma, when people are cut off from their gut sense, they become divorced from the vitality of the organic body. To foster greater emotional intelligence, it is necessary to open pathways of feeling into the viscera.

One of the ways we do this is by gently mobilizing the body through rocking, gliding, and spiral movements. This helps to stimulate the parasympathetic branch of the vagus nerve. Generally, when a movement regime is coupled with mindfulness-based practices that help track emotions in the body, it is possible to "wake up" areas that have been desensitized.

Many aspects of a yoga practice are designed to bring about such sensitivity. Dietary regulation, mindful breathing, *metta* practices (heart-centered meditations on loving-kindness), visualization, and postures (especially twists) help foster greater awareness in the gut. Another method to heal the internal organs, used by qigong and yoga practitioners alike, is to direct sound and vibration into individual organs.

Visceral Manipulation

The effects of āsana and prāṇāyāma on the viscera resemble the health benefits provided by visceral manipulation, an offshoot of osteopathic medicine. Jean-Pierre Barral and Pierre Mercier, in their seminal work on manual therapy for the viscera, describe the movement of the organs this way:

> This motion is an interdependent one because of serous membranes which envelop the organ, and the fasciae, ligaments and other living tissues which bind it to the rest of the organism. . . . All viscera should function properly, without any restrictions. Any restriction, fixation or adhesion to another structure, no matter how small, implies functional impairment of the organ. The consequent modification of its motion, repeated thousands of times daily in the body, can bring about significant changes, both to the organ itself and to any related structures.[7]

Certain yoga practices generate motility in the internal organs so that they function optimally. For instance, via a series of isolated abdominal movements called *kriyas,* techniques used for internal cleansing and purification, the gut is turned and swooshed like the spin cycle of a washing machine. When the abdominal organs are churned, it is essentially a kind of visceral manipulation.

The fascial compartments that surround and delineate the organ structures may compress, torque, or swell, and fibrotic tissue can amass in and around the viscera. Techniques such as *nauli* and uḍḍīyāna bandha help to break up adhesions within these connective tissues and aid in the irrigation of blood and lymph throughout the abdomal cavities. Changes in pressure in the connective tissues surrounding the abdominal organs can help reset metabolic rhythms related to cardiovascular, digestive, and endocrine function.

Uḍḍīyāna Bandha and the Liver

The effects of uḍḍīyāna bandha may best be observed in the liver. The liver, which contours to the underside of the diaphragm, includes the massive hepatic portal system that pulls blood upward from the small intestine, large intestine, stomach, pancreas, and spleen. The hepatic portal system is a highway of venous blood making its way back to the heart through the way station of the liver (the liver filters 1.5 liters of blood per minute, and 70 percent of that blood flows into the liver via the portal vein).[8] The role of the liver is immense and varied. It stores blood, forms plasma and proteins, metabolizes and stores nutrients, generates bile, and breaks down toxins. When the liver is sluggish, circulatory rhythms throughout the body are adversely affected, reducing ones prāṇic capacity. Uḍḍīyāna bandha works like a partial liver flush, as the muscular movement of the iliopsoas prompts a surge of blood through the hepatic portal vein into the liver, boosting the overall circulation of blood and lymph through the liver (see fig. 4.3).

PRACTICE

Squeezing the Abdominal Organs

The following setup places direct pressure on the abdominal organs in order to promote circulation through the gut.

Take a blanket and roll it up so that it is approximately four to six inches in circumference. Then stand with your feet as wide as your mat. Hold the blanket snug at the top of your thighs with your hands. Take a deep inhalation and with the exhalation, fold forward over the blanket roll. Meanwhile tuck the roll between your upper thighs and belly. As you fold into uttanāsana (standing forward bend) be sure that the wedged blanket puts direct pressure on your gut. If your hamstrings and spinal muscles are stiff, you may need to make the roll larger in order to trap it between the thighs and belly. Breathe into the prop and feel the local pressure on your abdominal organs. After a minute or more, take hold of the roll, press into your heels, and come up. Afterward, lay on your back and notice how your breath flows with greater ease into your abdomen.

Food, Nourishment, and the Intestinal Folds

In the gut, the intestines are compacted together in a confined space, in the way that the roots of a potted plant grow into the sides of its container. The gastrointestinal tract is approximately twenty-three feet (seven meters) in length, and it is compressed into an area the size of a twelve-inch mixing bowl. If you were to cut open the intestine and reveal its entire internal surface, that surface would be approximately as wide as a tennis court (including the doubles column). This extensive square footage suggests the importance of the intestine's role in maximizing the extraction of nutrients from the food we eat. The multiple folds within the alimentary canal enable the body to absorb the vital life-force, or prāṇa, encoded within the food.

The kinship between food and prāṇa plays a central role in the history of yogic thought and discipline. In the *Taittirīya Upaniṣad*, a collection of honorific verses to the forces of sun, wind, air, and water, several passages venerate food as the source of prāṇa. The following passage invokes the importance of food and what is referred to in yoga as the "food sheath" (*anna-maya-kośa*):

> Do not speak ill of food [*annaṃ*]. That shall be the rule. Life, verily, is food. The body is the eater of food. In life is the body established; life is established in the body. So is food established in food. He who knows that food is established in food, becomes established. He becomes an eater of food, possessing food. He becomes great in offspring and cattle and in the splendour of the sacred wisdom; great in fame.[9]

This revelatory passage praising food as the source of life speaks to the merits of establishing proper digestion. For it is through the assimilation of food that we build our blood, and blood is the primary carrier of oxygen and prāṇa. Without proper assimilation of nutritive matter from food into the bloodstream, the body cannot build its tissues. In Ayurvedic theory, the blood is formed from *rasa*, a semiliquid substance that is prepared in the digestive tract. Rasa is responsible for building muscle tissue, bone, fat, and marrow.[10] Building the food sheath through a balanced diet combined with good digestive capacity within the gastrointestinal tract is one of the primary means to fortify and heal the body.

The Belly Brain and the Cranial Brain

So far, we have examined the remarkable ways in which certain regions of the body mirror each other. This holds true for two critical bodily centers that play a role in the ingestion, assimilation, and processing of information—the belly brain and the cranial brain.

The third chakra, the belly chakra, and the sixth chakra, the cerebral chakra, share similarity in form and function (see figs. 4.3 and 7.5). In the way that the abdomen has wormlike folds of intestine compacted into a small space, the cranial cavity holds the brain's mass of convoluted folds. Like the small intestine, the potential surface area within the brain's convolutions is exponentially higher than is revealed on its exterior surface. If we were to unpack the brain, as we did the intestine, and spread open its interior corrugated folds and measure its inner surfaces, its total surface area would be approximately five times greater than its outer circumference. The potential for absorption in both the belly brain and the cranial brain far surpasses the limits of their actual shape.

The two brains are similar in that they are designed to absorb the maximum amount of information possible—the cranial brain registering perceptions, thoughts, memories, and emotions, and the belly brain soaking up nutritional input from food. Both brains employ a complex series of tasks to assimilate information and so operate via selective intelligence. Through electrical pulses, hormonal signals, and sensory receptors, the belly brain and cranial brain undergo complex decision-making processes.

The two brains undergo similar processes; they sift through, break down, and identify what can be used and what should be discarded. This process of identification and discrimination is critical for digesting the circumstances of a lifetime and for generating a sense of self.

Both brains have a capacity to recognize and remember a wide array of information.

It is safe to say that the two brains can be easily overwhelmed. When the brain is overwhelmed with information, it becomes blurry or fragmented. In the same way, strong feelings can besiege the gut leading to feelings of confusion and disorientation. When we are inundated by complex emotion, we experience feelings that are "too difficult to stomach"; symptoms may include nausea, indigestion, bloating, loss of appetite, irritable bowel syndrome (IBS), and light-headedness.

Digestion and the Primitive Worm

The digestive system is possibly the oldest system in the human body, predating the more sophisticated neurological, immunological, and hormonal systems. The human gastrointestinal (GI) tract harkens back to the cylindrical body of a worm, an invertebrate decomposer that ingests plant material through a mouthlike opening, has a gizzard that grinds down food, and an anus to eliminate. Earthworms have been active on this planet for 120 million years, and their fundamental digestive structure is an inherent part of our anatomy today. Simple nerve reflexes get relayed slowly through the worm body in very much the same way that nerve impulses pass between mouth and gut.

What makes human beings so complicated is that over and above this primitive digestive tube has evolved the "new brain," the rapid-fire neocortex. The reflexes and signals that are relayed in the gut are much slower than the high-speed connections made by the brain. For this reason it is easy for cognitive functioning to override the impulses that pass through the gut. When cognitive function overrides the slower digestive rhythms, the gut is prone to distress. This is due partly to disturbances of the delicate and complex vagus nerve that enervates the alimentary canal and internal organs. Emotional centers buried deep within the gut monitor feelings far below the radar of the rational brain. When in the throes of strong emotion, the rational brain, seeking control, dominates the "digestive brain" so that gut feelings that have real influence over the subtle body become thwarted, repressed, or ignored.

Personality and the Ecology of the Gut

Each of us is host to an entire parade of intestinal bacteria, such that billions of microbes inhabit our gut. These are microbes that we inherit from our parents and accumulate since childhood. Intestinal bacteria sift through, regulate, and catabolize the food we eat. The ecology of the gut is such an integral part of us that not only does it contribute to digestive function but it has real sway over the subtle body, affecting mood, attitude, and physical vitality. In the way that every single person is unique, the characteristic flora within our gut shapes who we are. Our temperamental disposition, our personality, and even our thinking are influenced by the microbial environment within our intestinal folds.

It is an ongoing challenge to balance the complex constitution of the gut, yet this is an essential task of the yogi. When the habitat of the microbial colonies is afflicted and there is poor intestinal flora, the prāṇa in the body cannot be sufficiently generated. In turn, this may inhibit overall concentration and meditative focus. There are numerous factors that weaken and disturb the microorganisms within the intestinal folds such as exposure to parasites, taking antibiotics, and eating poor food combinations. Yogis aim to create a harmonious environment within their gut via relaxation techniques, mindful eating, and supplemental probiotics.

The Intuitive Gut

What is unique and often overlooked is the abdominal brain's capacity to feel. Not only is the gut given the task of separating, organizing, and processing the food we ingest, but it also plays a significant role in sorting through thoughts, moods, perceptions, and emotions. The belly is a primary resource for intuition, processing information below or outside the radar of the cognitive mind. Yogic discipline along with other contemplative spiritual practices nurture an intuitive self. The English word *intuition* stems from the Latin root *intueri,* meaning to reflect on or contemplate. When we use our intuition, we reflect on that which we cannot see. This involves the gut sense, wherein moods, feelings, and premonitions pass in waves through the belly but are never made solid.

The belly brain, called the enteric nervous system, has the capacity to process independently of the cranial brain. Its capacity to self-regulate is still not fully understood even by experts in the field of gastroenterology. Yet we know that the gut operates at times without direct signaling from the central nervous system. In his book, *The Second Brain,* Michael Gershon describes the uniqueness of the belly brain:

> The enteric nervous system does not necessarily follow commands from the brain or spinal cord; nor does it inevitably send the information it receives back to them. The enteric nervous system can, when it chooses, process data its sensory receptors pick up all by themselves. . . . The enteric nervous system is thus not a slave of the brain but a contrarian, independent spirit. . . . It is a rebel, the only element of the peripheral nervous system that can elect not to do the bidding of the brain or spinal cord.[11]

In many regards, we are only vaguely aware of the intelligence of the belly brain. Its regulatory function occupies a kind of remote place in our field of sensitivity, yet we have numerous references in the language that point to it, expressions such as "gut instinct," "gut reaction," and "spill your guts."

Intuition is a means to connect to the substratum of the unconscious. It links us to dreams and the unspoken, like a hand reaching out to mystery. Through deep, internal listening and by exploring the threshold places—between inhalation and exhalation, night and day, sun and moon, real and imaginary—we connect to a sense of intuition. Within the stillness of meditation or in the experience of yoga nidrā (a state of awareness that hovers between wakefulness and sleep), we attune to the elusive realm of spirit.

The Dan Tian

Midway between the navel and the pelvic floor is a gravitational center called the *dan tian.* In Taoist practices and in the martial arts, the dan tian is a reservoir of chi and a source of vitality. Directing awareness into the dan tian complements the powerful upward surge of uḍḍīyāna bandha emphasized in yoga training.

Anatomically, the dan tian is located along the embankment of the inner pelvis, at the lower end of the iliopsoas complex. Tai chi practitioners and meditation masters use this low center of gravity, like the ballast of a boat, to establish weight and stability. It is said in the Tao Te Ching that the root of all lightness is heaviness, and thus settling into the dan tian provides both anatomical and psychological composure.

The Chinese expression *dan tian* refers to a "field" (*tian*) of "fluid vitality" (*dan*) that dwells like an underground lake at the base of the spine. In the depth of meditation, awareness should descend into the basin of the belly in the way that mist settles over a valley. This downward settling is complemented by opening in the third lumbar vertebra (L3) called the Gate of Life (in Chinese, *ming men*). The Gate of Life is an acupressure point in TCM that supports the kidney essence and is integral to the body's defensive chi (see figs. 2.8 and 5.2).

Thus, resting in the dan tian brings about fluid awareness. It also enables one to remain grounded in the face of adversity. It is by residing in the lower dan tian that martial artists can resist being thrown, knocked over, or otherwise put down. One of my teachers once described the strength of the dan tian as a means by which "nothing can knock you off the center of your day."

◈

Lowrider Āsana

There is a cultural phenomenon where I live in Santa Fe, New Mexico, that demonstrates the value of a low center of gravity. On Friday nights along the streets of San Francisco, Alameda, and Guadalupe (small two-lane roads that circle the historic downtown plaza in Santa Fe), young, local Latino men with their jeans slung low on their hips and their caps turned backward creep along in their souped-down cars. They drive refurbished Camaros and Mustangs or the old family Buick with new paint jobs, white-walled tires, tinted windows, and "No Fear" stickers in the rear windows. They set the carriage of their lowriders such that they hover inches off the street, requiring a pace slower than a crawl, a kind of antispeed, which confounds the summer tourists hustling to their dinner reservations. The boom of their stereos, a thumping pulse so low it vibrates the lowest chakras down to the perineum, resounds in the summer night. The attitude of the driver and passenger always says simply, "This is where it's at."

I call it the "lowrider āsana," and it suggests the value of rooting down, keeping a low center of gravity, and moving slowly. The message is, be cool, don't flare up. The steadiness of the lowrider crawl and its ground-level presence speaks to the realm in the body that masters of the internal arts rely on for power and composure, the lower dan tian.

The Navel Chakra

The navel plays such an esteemed role in the body. Not only is it the link to the vital breath—the blood—that comes from the mother but it is located near the gravitational center of our being. In yoga, the navel is considered to be its own chakra, called the *nābhi chakra,* another name for maṇipūra chakra. In the third chapter of Patañjali's Yoga Sutras, dedicated to yoga *siddhis* (powers), is a verse dedicated to the navel chakra *(nābhi cakre kāya vyūha jnāñam* III.29). This verse suggests that the navel is the hub, the spiritual pivot of the body, and like a flash drive, contains knowledge of the body's internal systems.

It is valuable to reflect on the idea that all movement originates in the navel. If we consider the flexed curl of the posture of a newborn (the shape of child's pose), we can imagine how the belly button is the nucleus for future postural development. The navel initiates extension of the legs, arms, and neck—movement patterns first actualized by the fetus in utero. In her groundbreaking work on somatic organization, Bonnie Bainbridge Cohen refers to this umbilicus center as "navel radiation" and compares the navel to the center point of a starfish, whose limbs extend outward from its primary center.

PRACTICE

Centering into the Dan Tian

The following exercises help establish a feeling of space, ease, and stability in the lower abdomen. Each exercise is designed to gather and contain the abdominal chi so as to embody the serenity of deep, still water.

Assume the horse stance, a primary qigong position, by standing with your feet slightly wider than hip-width apart. Allow the weight of your body to sink into the ground and spread through the bones of your feet. Sense an internal balance, a natural and harmonious stance. Bend your knees slightly so the backs of your knees are soft. At the same time, allow your tailbone to drop as you settle into your lower abdomen. In dan tian breathing, the lower back and the lower belly should expand. Allow your breath to seep into the depths of your abdomen as if you are watering a plant. Observe the expansion of your kidneys as they broaden away from each other and sense a relaxed vitality in the region of the ming men, the Gate of Life. With each exhalation, root downward into your feet and pelvis. The texture of your breath should be *jing, chang,* and *xi*—"tranquil, long, and fine." Now hold your hands in front of your lower abdomen as though you are holding a small pot. Bring your awareness to the empty container formed by your hands and fill the imaginary vessel with chi or breath. The diameter of the vessel can change, but concentrate on bringing relaxed, ample breath between your hands that symbolize the dan tian. Stay for five to ten minutes.

Next, lie on your back with your knees bent and your feet flat on the floor directly under your knees. Re-create a similar wide-brimmed feeling in your lower abdomen. With your elbows bent, rest your fingertips on the region just below your navel. Feel your breath infuse into your lower spine and abdomen. Visualize a hollow opening within your navel, like a small sinkhole in the sand. Sense a connection from your superficial navel to the underlying fibers an inch below your navel. Imagine the depths of your navel sinking into wet sand, such that your entire abdomen softens and widens. Become aware of the way your navel refers all the way back to the front of your spine. Continue this process of dropping inward for ten minutes.

5

THE DIAPHRAGM

The Prāṇa Pump

When we practice our mind always follows our breathing. When we inhale, the air comes into the inner world. When we exhale the air goes out to the outer world. The inner world is limitless, the outer world is also limitless. We say "inner world" or "outer world" but actually there is just one whole world.

—Shunryu Suzuki, *Zen Mind, Beginner's Mind*[1]

In the ascent from the plantar surface of the foot to the crown of the head, the climb through the third chakra in the belly to the fourth chakra located in the heart is particularly arduous. Here we must pass from the "belly of the beast," with its personal, gut sense of *me*, to the heart, with its transpersonal sense of *we*. Empathetic resonance is the intention of the *bodhisattva* who, in the Buddhist faith, vows to nurture the well-being of all. In the energy of the chakras, this transition from the self-centered will of the third chakra to the heart of inclusivity suggests a move to a wider, more spacious and humane view.

When addressing the question of personal self, one of my Zen teachers Roshi Joan Sutherland would ask her students, "How open is your sense of self? What are the boundaries of self? How permeable is it?" When the shackles that constrain the sense of *I* are loosened, self-identity becomes less confined and more inclusive. This view in Zen training is sometimes referred to as Big Mind, which could also be thought of as Big Heart. The transition across the diaphragm to the abode of the heart evokes this move.

This chapter maps this transition and describes the essential role the diaphragm plays as the regulator of respiration and prāṇa. It is impossible to define prāṇa; any attempt to explain it is akin to trying to explain the meaning of God. To say that prāṇa is simply the breath that flows in and out of the lungs is too limiting. All the systems of the body—the nervous, digestive, reproductive, and endocrine—are sustained by the movement of prāṇa. Prāṇa has a fluid quality. The pulsating rhythms of the breath can be felt throughout every cell and synapse in the body. All fascia in the body move reciprocally with the diaphragm, as the diaphragm is the primary fulcrum for conducting kinetic flow through the body. In this sense the diaphragm governs inherent motion in the body, and changes within the respiratory rhythm have repercussions on the health and organization of all bodily tissues. This chapter explores the structural location of the diaphragm and its function as the prime mover of prāṇa in yoga discipline. We will see how the motion of the diaphragm is prone to restriction due to postural and emotional tension.

The Diaphragm: The Great Divide

In the body there is a marked change across the barrier of the diaphragm, from the crowded abdominal cavern below to the "higher ground" of the heart and lung above it. Below the diaphragm the organs and their associated nerves are responsible for digestion, blood building, storage, and cleanup, whereas the lungs and heart above the diaphragm are responsible for oxygenating and circulating the blood. To understand the considerable differences between these two partitioned spaces, it is helpful to compare the torso to an eighteenth-century clipper ship.

In the clipper ship, the deck divides the hull below from the masts and sails above deck. Sometimes called the "weather deck" or "shelter deck," it is a threshold that separates two worlds. Below the ship's main deck, in darkened spaces within the hull, are a series of quarters and compartments that provide order, storage, and fuel for the ship. In a similar way the abdominal organs, compartmentalized below the diaphragm, process, sort, assimilate, and store fuel for the body. Beneath the deck of the clipper ship, the bilge was used for evacuating seawater (which translates to the bladder's job in the body), the cargo to store supplies (the liver and kidneys), the stokehold for the ship's furnace (the small intestine), and the kitchen for feeding the crew (the stomach). The bustle of activity in the ship's hull kept the vessel in good working order. This industrious activity was necessary for the ship's daily maintenance in the way that the churn of digestion sustains the body.

The routine task of a sailor sailing across the Atlantic from Europe to America was to adjust the stays and reposition the sails according to shifts in the prevailing winds. In prāṇāyāma, we make similar adjustments to our spine, ribs, and diaphragm to catch the gusts of inhalation or release tension on the exhalation. In the way that a ship's captain would continuously monitor trade winds to navigate the open ocean, prāṇāyāma requires ongoing sensitivity and observation to track changes in pressure, velocity, and tension within the lung tissue (fig. 5.1).

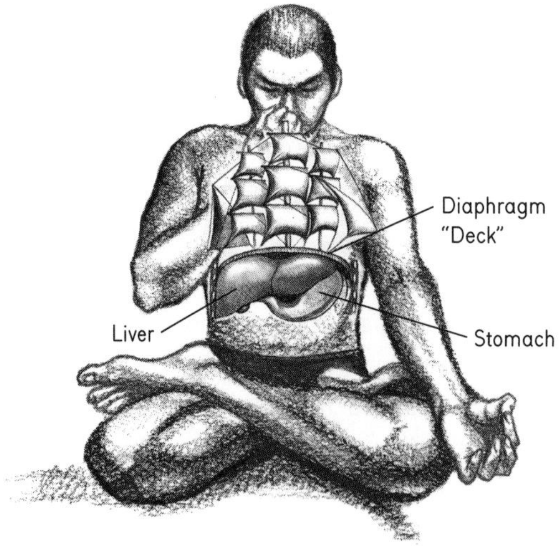

Figure 5.1 The Sails of the Lungs in Prāṇāyāma

The Conscious Breather

Cardiac and pulmonary output within the thoracic cavity can be modulated in ways impossible in the abdominal cavity. While the rhythmic beat of the lungs and heart does not require conscious prompting by voluntary musculature, it is possible to manipulate the filling and narrowing phases of the lung tissue. Intentional altering of the breath will impart immediate changes to cardiovascular rhythm. Restraint (yama) of the breath (prāṇā) involves arresting the breath in a variety of ways. Breath retention has subtle yet potent effects on circulatory rhythms, neurological activity, and cerebral function. Thus, above the diaphragm and within the chest cavity and the heart chakra, we encounter a more conscious or higher level of order than is possible within the purely autonomic churnings of the gut.

This possibility defines the practice of prāṇāyāma, the fourth limb of Aṣṭāṇga Yoga. Temporarily suspending the breath is preparatory for further concentration practices that impart subtle shifts within the flow of awareness (dhāraṇā, dhyāna, and samādhi). In Patañjali's Yoga Sutras one of the verses defining prāṇāyāma states that prāṇāyāma "dissolves the covering that veils the light of awareness" (*tataḥ kṣīyate prakāśa āvaraṇam* II.52). This implies that altered respiratory rhythm has a profound effect on consciousness. By removing the covering that obscures awareness, awareness can "shine" (*prakāśa*). In the Eight-Limbed Yoga of Patañjali, the luminosity and clarity that prāṇāyāma manifests are attributable to both heart and mind. In any case, the ability to manipulate the breath is unique to humankind and sets us apart from the animal kingdom (imagine your dog or cat lying on the kitchen floor practicing prāṇāyāma!).

The Crux of the Spine: The Lumbodorsal Hinge

The transition between the lumbar and thoracic spine is a critical juncture and marks the divide between the lower and upper halves of the body. This region is an epicenter for all biological activity. At the lumbodorsal hinge—the juncture of the twelfth thoracic and first lumbar vertebra (T12-L1)—respiratory, circulatory, hormonal, digestive, and musculoskeletal systems converge. The lumbodorsal hinge is where the posterior curvature of the thoracic spine becomes the anterior curve of the lumbar spine. At this juncture, the spine is endowed with its greatest capacity for spring.

We saw previously how transitions in spinal curvature can be tricky in the case of the anterior lumbar curve changing course and becoming the posterior sacral curve. The lumbodorsal hinge is a transition in the vertebral column where spinal mechanics often become derailed. This area can be too loose, as in the tendency toward lordosis (an overarched spine), or it can become compact and dense, as when the dorsal hinge collapses and the lumbar curvature is reversed (slumpasana).

This region incorporates the solar plexus. The solar plexus is analogous to a lesser-known chakra, the *sūrya chakra,* located just below the diaphragm. The sūrya (sun) chakra is veritably the only chakra that gets directly translated into English. The solar plexus is the hearth of the body, home to the *samāna vāyu,* which translates as "equalizing wind current." It is the intermediary region of the body between the low-lying *apāna vāyu,* centered in the pelvis, and the upper wind called the *prāṇa vāyu,* located in the heart and lungs. The solar plexus is the seat of *pitta,* where digestive fire burns hottest. It serves as the body's engine, providing

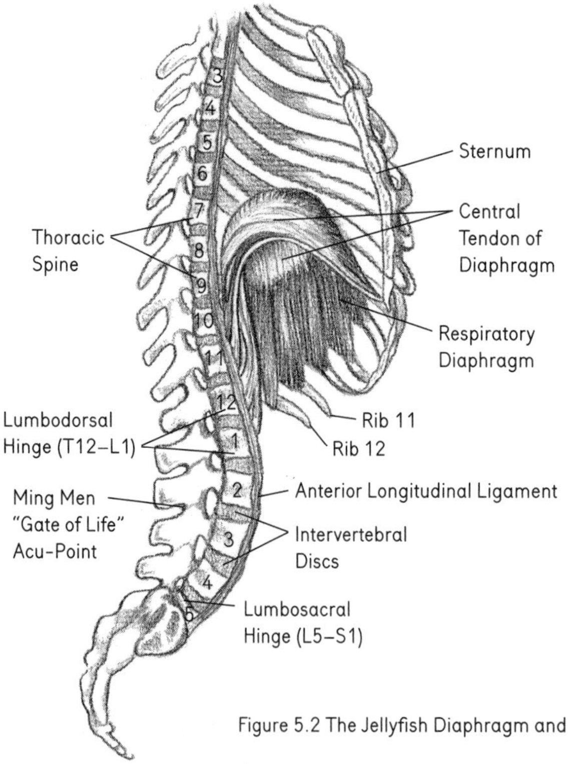

Figure 5.2 The Jellyfish Diaphragm and the Lumbodorsal Hinge

sustained energy and metabolic endurance for the entire body. In both yoga and traditional Chinese medicine, this area relates to the fire element and is likened to a furnace that provides steady fuel for the body. In qigong this furnace is referred to as "the golden stovepipe," a striking analogy for the heat and intensity generated in the solar plexus.

PRACTICE

Balancing the Lumbodorsal Hinge

This practice helps bring awareness to the lumbodorsal junction, the attachments of the diaphragm, and the *ming men*, the Gate of Life point. This sequence of poses will help balance the transition in your spine between the lumbar and thoracic curves.

Begin standing in taḍāsana (mountain pose) and loop a belt over your lower ribs so that it is located below your sternum and above your navel. Do not make the strap too tight, but make it fit so that when you take a full inhalation you can feel your lower ribs and upper abdomen expand outward against the prop. Stand with your feet hip-width apart and plant your feet firmly on the floor. Take several rhythmic breaths, expanding your ribs against the strap at the level of your lumbodorsal junction (T12-L1). Then raise your arms into *ūrdhva hastāsana* (extended arm pose) so that your hands are shoulder-width apart. Avoid overarching your ribs and spine forward into the "dismount āsana." If this happens you will overextend at the lumbodorsal hinge and your ribs will push forward like an arching gymnast seeking a score of 10 from the judges. Maintain tadāsana and breathe into your side and back ribs, using the presence of the strap to assess balance.

Then keeping the strap on, sweep your arms forward to the floor and step back into downward dog. Adjust the tension on the strap as needed and once again direct your breath into your floating ribs (Rib 11–12) and diaphragm at the level of the lumbodorsal hinge (fig. 5.2). Again, avoid overarching your spine, which will cause your ribs and chest to collapse toward the floor. Feel your ribs expand against the strap and at the same time do the dog tilt (anterior tilt) in your pelvis as described in chapter 2.

Then come to sit in virāsana (pose of virility) with the belt still around you. Breathe into your lower trunk at the level of the strap and imagine your breath contacting the ming men point at your second lumbar vertebra. Maintain the concave curvature of your lumbar spine and the posterior curve of your thoracic spine. At the lumbodorsal hinge actively stretch your spine upward toward your crown. Visualize orienting your entire torso and skull from your lumbodorsal hinge. Stay for several minutes before lying down to release your spine in śavāsana.

Under the Hood of the Diaphragm

The diaphragm is held firmly in place by the organs that surround it. It is sandwiched between the liver, stomach, kidneys, and spleen below and the heart and lungs above. The diaphragm orchestrates movement of all thoracic and abdominal viscera. Seven organs attach directly to the diaphragm: the lungs, heart (and pericardium), stomach, liver, kidneys, spleen, and pancreas. Of course the organs are not free-floating in the body. If they were, the liver could end up on the pelvic floor and the lung could slide up into the ear. The organs are attached to each other and to the diaphragm via ligaments. If the organs are healthy and unrestricted in their motility, they will slide against one another as part of an orchestrated wobble. Should one of the organs be caught or snagged by tension in its enveloping tissues, the movement of the diaphragm may alter as it accommodates the strain. Healthy organs should glide fluidly and smoothly over one another like a basket full of fresh-caught fish.

The organs below the diaphragm are held in place via natural suction. In order for the diaphragm to move in its fullest possible range, there must be balanced tension in the solar plexus below the diaphragm and in the thoracic cavity above. The diaphragm is always moving in response to positive and negative pressures between the abdomen and the chest. Under the diaphragm, two possible scenarios can impair the fluid movement of breathing. One is ptosis, or prolapse, wherein an organ inferior to the diaphragm droops or pulls away from the diaphragm. The other is hypertension, wherein the organs and surrounding fascia tighten and pin upward against the diaphragm, like an escaped helium balloon trapped against the ceiling.

When we stand, the abdominal organs and diaphragm are subject to a certain degree of pressure. People who stand for long periods of time are prone to shallow breathing and dramatic changes in blood pressure due to the way the lumbodorsal hinge, abdominal viscera, and respiratory diaphragm compress. However, when we are supine (or prone), the pull on the diaphragm is reduced, the visceral ligaments relax, and the normal excursion of the breath is longer. For this reason, sleep rejuvenates the organic body by allowing the abdominal organs and adjoining vessels to decompress. When learning yogic breathing, it is best to learn prāṇāyāma in a reclined position (ideally with the back propped on blankets or a bolster) to release pressure built up in the abdomen, expand the chest, and maximize the diaphragm's range of motion.

During inhalation, the diaphragm moves inferiorly causing the organs to depress downward and expand forward. As a result, the belly expands. The abdomen's capacity to balloon outward supports the process of natural diaphragmatic breathing. When an infant or child breathes, his or her belly distends forward like the belly of a tai chi master. Unfortunately, for many adults, the natural wavelike movement of the diaphragm is inhibited. This may be due to trauma of some kind whereby the upper gut and muscular diaphragm get caught in a startle response—what Thomas Hanna coined the "red-light reflex." This protective reflex causes the ventral side of the body to contract and cower. Chronic abdominal tension blocks the natural and appropriate forward protrusion of the abdomen on inhalation and alters the smooth orchestration of the diaphragm during breathing.

PRACTICE

Noticing Respiratory Constriction

The following series of observations involve noticing how stress affects respiration. In yoga we use our bodies as a laboratory to research physiological change, and this practice requires being mindful of respiratory tension off the mat. The next time that you experience a rush of anxiety or fear, carefully observe the way stress affects your abdominal organs and diaphragm. In particular, notice the organs and connective tissues just below the hood of your diaphragm. Do these organs clench or tighten? How does it affect your inhalation? Can you feel your respiratory diaphragm constrict? Do you notice compression in your pelvic floor?

Although it is difficult to gain sensitivity in the midst of distress, observe changes in your respiratory rhythm as best as you can. When you attempt to inhale, is your breath choppy and broken? Does your upper chest feel tight? Notice any constriction around your eyes, jaw, tongue, and throat. Note any changes in your blood pressure. Should your blood pressure elevate, it may prove more difficult to draw the inhalation into your body. Even if you tell yourself to relax and take the proverbial deep breath, tension in the diaphragm does not easily subside. It takes time for an emotional charge to dissipate and for the respiratory rhythm to return to normal.

This entire process requires keen inward listening. Typically students of yoga spend time in mindful breathing only when their breath is passive and relaxed. Maintaining subjective awareness in the midst of difficulty off the mat requires real attentiveness as constrictive states cause distraction and confusion. Over time, by generating awareness during states of stress, it is less likely that agitation will overwhelm your nervous system.

The Pelvic and Respiratory Polar Caps

In our map of the horizontal diaphragms of the body, the respiratory diaphragm is the third horizontal. It correlates with the first two broad, sling-like structures that we have already reviewed—one at the sole of the foot and the other at the pelvic floor. As we have seen, congestion, rigidity, or laxity in any one of these planes can impair movement in the other diaphragms. Since we stand on two legs, our aim in yoga practice is to move from the ground upward, initially gaining elasticity and responsiveness within the plantar fascia at the sole of the foot.

The sphere-like space of the abdomen can be compared to a globe. The northern cap of the globe is the respiratory diaphragm and the southern cap is the perineum. Both structures have central tendons—tough fibrous weaves at the center of the "polar caps" that orient and reinforce the diaphragms. In all yoga postures, we align these two caps in order to facilitate a more prolonged, uninhibited breath. The dynamic tension between these two poles in part determines efficiency in breathing. When the lower pole of the pelvic diaphragm is positioned directly under the upper pole of the respiratory diaphragm, breathing is easier (see B of fig 5.3). When the two diaphragms are misaligned, the tensions within the pelvic and abdominal cavities compete and breathing may be compromised (see A and C of fig. 5.3).

In haṭha yoga, the compatibility of these two diaphragms is critical, especially during prāṇāyāma when movements within the spine, rib basket, and abdominal muscles are subtle. (I prefer rib "basket" to rib "cage," for the weave of a wicker basket better resembles the plaiting of intercostal muscles between the ribs.)

PRACTICE

Breathing into the Abdominopelvic Balloon

This exercise helps to coordinate the movement of the pelvic and respiratory diaphragms in breathing. Assume a comfortable seated position, either virāsana (pose of virility), sukhāsana (contentment pose), or siddhāsana (accomplished pose) and support your sitting bones on a four- to six-inch lift of blankets or bolster. Lift your spine so that you align your head, chest, and pelvis. Orient your trunk so that your pelvic floor

Figure 5.3 Orientation of Respiratory and Pelvic Diaphragms

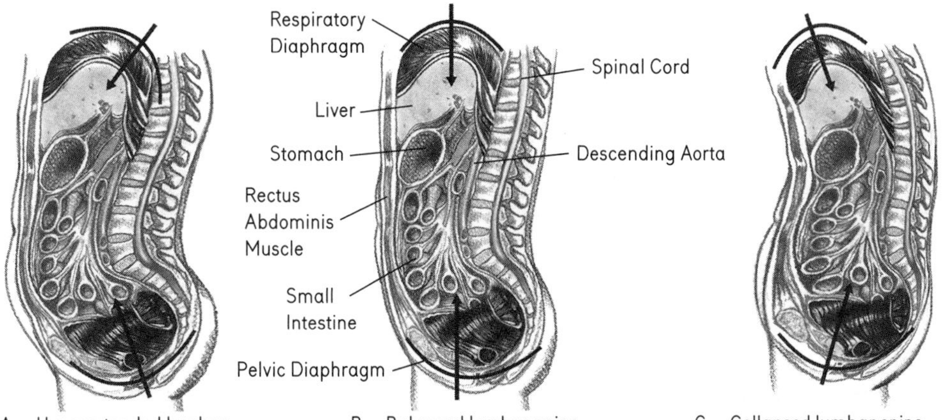

A—Hyperextended lumbar spine with disorganized pelvic and respiratory diaphragms

B—Balanced lumbar spine with harmonious pelvic and respiratory diaphragms

C—Collapsed lumbar spine with disorganized pelvic and respiratory diaphragms diaphragm and respiratory diaphragm align like the north and south polar caps of the globe.

Without collapsing your spine, relax the sidewalls of your abdomen and allow your belly to spread laterally. Avoid gripping your rectus abdominis, the muscle along the front of your belly that runs from pubic bone to sternum. Release any tension that may be harbored in the muscular sheath of your respiratory diaphragm. As you inhale fill your lungs and feel your abdominal balloon enlarge. Note the way your respiratory diaphragm descends as the circumference of your abdomen expands. First expand the upper belly, then expand downward to the level of the dan tian below your navel. Expand the globe of your abdomen in such a way that you gain breadth and space throughout your abdominopelvic cavity.

Next imagine you are blowing up a balloon inside your abdomen, inflating it all the way down to your pelvic floor. Your perineum should act as a tie to this balloon. At the very end of each exhalation, secure the tie (that is, perform mūla bandha) by lifting your pelvic floor. As you breathe in, your pelvic floor will drop slightly given the expansion of the abdominopelvic balloon. Observe how your pelvic and respiratory diaphragms move in synchrony—the base of the balloon at the perineum should follow the upward and downward flow of the respiratory diaphragm. Practice for five to ten minutes before lying down in śavāsana to rest.

PRACTICE

Helium Dog Pose

This practice invites you to feel the parallel movements between your pelvic floor and respiratory diaphragms. Take adho mukha śvānāsana (downward-facing dog pose). Step your feet apart so your stance is the width of your mat. This will encourage your sitting bones, sacrum, and pelvic floor to widen and spread. As you press firmly into your hands, elongate the sides of your trunk. Press your thighbones back in order to lengthen your side waist and lumbar spine. Then lift your heels upward by sinking your weight into the mound of your big toe and of your little toe (front two corners of the foot). At the same time pitch your sitting bones upward so that both your heels and sitting bones elevate off the floor. This will encourage a forward tilt, or "dog tilt" in your pelvis. Expand your breath into the lateral margins of your abdomen and feel a horizontal spreading across your midback. Avoid simply pulling or pressing your abdomen back toward your spine. Rather allow it to rise and spread as if you have a hot air balloon

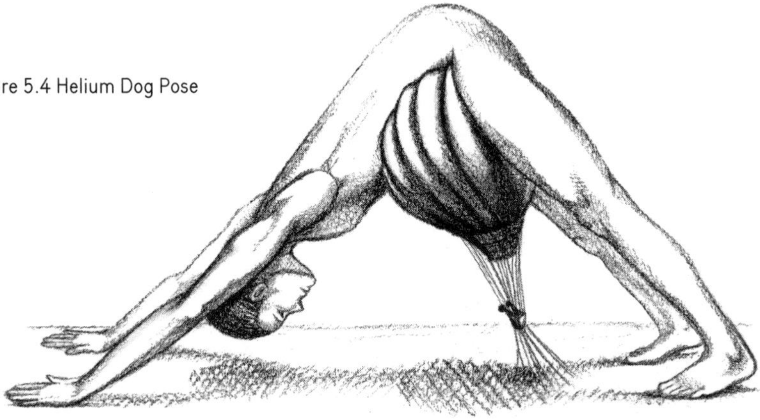

Figure 5.4 Helium Dog Pose

aloft in the space of your abdomen. Feel the way the imagined helium balloon provides buoyancy and support for your lower spine and abdominal organs. Stay for two minutes (fig. 5.4).

The Jellyfish Diaphragm

The architecture of the respiratory diaphragm is often misunderstood. For practitioners of the internal arts, a clear understanding of the anatomy of breathing is valuable, for it helps us discern greater nuance and inflection within the breath. If the perception of the diaphragm is ill-conceived, it can undermine any attempt to articulate, refine, and gain greater sensitivity for the tempo and cadence of the breath. I have found that the practice of prāṇāyāma is greatly enhanced by an understanding of the inherent motion of the respiratory diaphragm.

The diaphragm is not a flat muscular disk, in the shape of a Frisbee that separates the abdomen from the thorax. Its structure is more like a dome or hood (see fig 5.2). Its muscular fibers are nearly as long vertically as they are wide. Perhaps the best way to visualize and sense the diaphragm is to imagine the body of a jellyfish.

Not long ago I took my six-year-old to the Monterey Bay Aquarium, a living museum of Pacific sealife along the California coast. My son was enamored by the sea otter display and shark tank, but I was awestruck by the jellyfish exhibit, featuring ghostlike hoods of tissue that resemble floating diaphragms. Jellyfish have been on our planet for more than 650 million years. They are ancient boneless shrouds with membranous and translucent bodies (uplit in day-glo colors in the aquarium tanks). In the ocean they suspend like mini space capsules, their umbrella-like hoods billowing in the current. In the human body the pliable edges of our respiratory diaphragm rise and fall like the undulating tissue of the jellyfish.

The jellyfish glides through water via alternating rhythms of contraction and expansion. It does not have a nervous system; it simply moves in response to the tidal flows around it. The human diaphragm is also subject to fluid tempos relating to blood pressure and circulatory rhythms. The heartbeat, the spleen beat, the kidney beat, the liver pulse, and the contractile rhythms of the stomach all influence breathing and the pumping mechanism of the diaphragm.

When we breathe, the excursion of the diaphragm's rigid center is minimal. Rather, the diaphragm's elastic outer rim moves, lifting and descending with each breath. Certain prāṇāyāma techniques are designed to stretch the diaphragm and make its outer edges more elastic. The prāṇāyāma breath *kapālabhāti* (skull shining breath) rapidly pumps the diaphragm so it swiftly expands and contracts like a bellows. This "Breath of Fire" stretches the muscular fibers at the lateral margins of the diaphragm, where it attaches to the inside wall of the ribs. While exercising the respiratory diaphragm, the Breath of Fire prompts a surge of blood and lymph throughout the abdominal organs.

PRACTICE

Floating the Diaphragm

This exercise makes the fibers of the respiratory diaphragm more elastic and brings greater sensitivity to the muscular slips at the periphery of the diaphragm.

Assume a comfortable seated position so that your lower spine is supported and your side waist is lifted away from your pelvis. Begin by relaxing your tongue and jaw and breathe slowly and softly in order to sense the natural rhythm of your breath. Bring your awareness to your midtrunk and release any clenching or gripping in your diaphragm. Try to draw your inhalation into the lower lobes of your lungs. This will help increase the expansion of your middle ribs in such a way that your rib basket moves outward and upward. Sense the edges of your diaphragm expanding and contracting like the gelatinous form of the jellyfish. Note in figure 5.2 where the edges of your diaphragm attach to your ribs, spine, and sternum. Maintain firmness in your spine while allowing the edges of your diaphragm to "float." Visualize your diaphragm drawing downward on each inhalation as your lungs inflate. On each exhalation, allow your diaphragm to waft back up toward its domed position. Continue this breathing exploration for ten minutes.

Asymmetrical Breathing and the Double-Domed Diaphragm

While the extremities of the arms and legs are bilaterally symmetrical (barring patterns of strain that occur over the course of a lifetime), the organic body from the neck to the pelvic floor is asymmetrical. This asymmetry results in the body's unique intrinsic motion and determines the irregular motion of the respiratory diaphragm. The motion of breathing is, in a word, wonky.

The muscle of the respiratory diaphragm is not symmetrical. It is double-domed with two hemispheres, the right dome being larger and higher than the left one. It is classified as a single muscle, because the contractile fibers that form the left and right domes converge onto the powerful fibrous complex of the central tendon. However, it is not too far-fetched to say that we have two diaphragms. For students of the internal arts, this has interesting correlations, given the body's two lungs, two nostrils, and two sides of the brain. A skilled practitioner schooled in the art of prāṇāyāma can, to some extent, isolate the movements of the right and left domes of the diaphragm. Alternate nostril breathing (*nāḍī śodhana*) plays a role in this, as the right nostril correlates to the right dome of the diaphragm and the left nostril to the left dome; if you look in the mirror at your "double-domed" nostrils, you can imagine how they are paired to the hemispheres of your diaphragm.

I suggest that the diaphragm is both double and singular. This may have interesting parallels to the nature of consciousness itself. We have already seen how in classical yoga the breath is intimately linked to consciousness. Consciousness may be considered singular, undifferentiated, or nondual (suggested by the powerful notion of *brāhman* in the Vedānta tradition) yet plural in its capacity to identify and reflect a multiplicity of things. Much could be said about the dynamic of the singular and dual in terms of the wisdom teachings, but for the moment, let's stay with the anatomical structure of the diaphragm. At the end of this chapter, I will explore the paradox of breathing and how this paradox relates to consciousness.

The right dome of the diaphragm rises above the left dome. This is due to the mass and girth of the liver nestled directly underneath the right hood. In terms of the subtle body, the right hemisphere of the diaphragm and the liver, gall bladder, and right lung correlate to the active (yang) fire channel in the body known as the piṅgalā or sūrya nāḍī. The left dome of the diaphragm and the stomach, pancreas, spleen, and left lung correspond to the receptive (yin) channel known as the *idā* or *chandra nāḍī*.

Above the diaphragm, the heart in situ is also asymmetrical, positioned slightly left of the midline (see fig. 6.7). When we refer to the heart in yoga, we often refer to the mystical or spiritual heart that we imagine residing in the center chest. Anatomically, the heart is shifted left, contributing to the asymmetrical pairing of the two diaphragms wherein the left side of the diaphragm is lower. As a result, the left lung is slightly smaller than the right. Correspondingly, the left lung has only two lobes, whereas the right lung has three lobes. The right and left bronchi, like flexible corrugated vacuum hoses, fork off the trachea and penetrate into each lung. They are also asymmetrical—the right bronchus is stouter and thicker than the left, because the traction of the right lung is stronger than that of the left lung.

This helps explain why the motion of the inherent breath wave is not symmetrical but more like a wobble. The overall fluctuating rhythm determines the diastole and systole movement of the cardiac cycle. It is important to note that the heart is not the only organ that beats: each of the organs in the body has a pulse and goes through a pumping motion (motility). The organic expansion and contraction of any one organ is synchronized with the pump-like motion of the other organs. Together the organs pulse in symphonic rhythm. The individual "beats" play off each other in a kind of arrhythmic pattern that creates the overall wobble. Blood pressure, hormonal activity, and stimulation of the nervous system (combined with many other factors) also affect the orchestration of these interrelated rhythms. In addition to the lopsided movement of the organs, any history of trauma or repetitive strain, especially in one shoulder, one side of the ribs, or neck, may contribute to respiratory asymmetry.

PRACTICE

Nāḍīs, Nostrils, and the Double-Domed Diaphragm

This meditation will help delineate and refine the movement of your diaphragm when breathing. You'll feel the side of your diaphragm and determine which side presents more of a barrier and which moves with greater ease.

Assume a comfortable seated position with your pelvis raised on a three- to six-inch-high support. Sit so your back is firm and your front body is lifted and receptive. Sense the sturdy muscular flap of your diaphragm spanning the middle of your trunk. Begin with a slow and soft natural rhythm of breath. Bring your awareness to the flow of breath through your right nostril. How open is your right nostril? Then bring sensitivity to your liver and diaphragm on the right side of your chest. How does your right diaphragm move relative to your liver as you breathe in? Does your liver provide a real barrier to the downward excursion of your diaphragm? Does the tug on your right diaphragm feel different at all from the movement of your left diaphragm? This right side relates to the solar channel of the body, the sūrya or piṅgalā nāḍī.

Now focus your awareness on your left nostril as it correlates to the left dome of your diaphragm. How open is your left nostril? Is it more or less open than your right?

Observe the downward excursion of the left side of your diaphragm on inhalation as it moves against your stomach. This relates to the lunar channel of your body (idā or chandra nāḍī). Now compare the two sides of your diaphragm again. Does one side move with greater ease than the other side? Notice the slight wobble in the inhalation phase of your breath. Most likely you will feel greater restriction on your right side, given the relative density of the liver. Typically the motion of the left side has more ease, because the organ of the stomach on the left is hollow and more distensible. Given that the stomach is more expandable, the left-side ribs often protrude slightly forward of the right lower ribs.

Continue with this exploration in breathing for five to ten minutes.

At the Altar of the Diaphragm

Prāṇa, the animating force in the body, is activated primarily by the movement of the respiratory diaphragm. Via the expansion and contraction of the diaphragm, all tissues in the body are enlivened and sustained. Thus, the diaphragm is the centerpiece of the body whose movement sparks life into every fiber, cell, and synapse. Given the sacredness of prāṇa in yoga, the diaphragm could be thought of as a living altar. Rather than a fixed and static platform, this altar is in perpetual motion. Its movements, along with those of the organs and vessels that intersect it, are continuous and cooperative. Its dynamic pump-like action is the very basis of life. In Sanskrit this life-generating expansion and contraction is called *spanda*, a pulse that is necessary for all life.

In the Catholic tradition, the altar is an elevated structure or dais upon which the Eucharist, the "original sacrifice," is re-created. On the dais, a strange and wonderful alchemical process uniting spirit and matter is set in motion. We have already seen how the process of yoga comes about through alchemical changes in the body and mind. The Catholic faith believes in a similar alchemy called transubstantiation, wherein bread becomes the body of Christ and wine symbolizes his blood. In the human body, the altar of the respiratory diaphragm is the site where prāṇa undergoes an alchemical process whereby oxygen from the air is diffused into the blood and is transported to all living tissues. The magical thing about breathing is that, with every breath, this alchemy occurs over and over again. Thus, the word *respiration* suggests not only the intake of breath but the recurrent pathway of spirit.

The prāṇa is a gift that keeps on giving and a source of boundless joy. Prāṇa is auspicious; to be born into a precious human existence (a term used by Tibetan meditation teachers) is to be blessed with this animating force. Many passages from the earliest yoga teachings exalt prāṇa as a means to realize this joy. In the subtle body, when one abides in the joy of prāṇa, it is called the *ānanda-maya-kośa,* or "sheath of bliss." In the *Taittirīya Upaniṣad* the body of bliss is described this way, "For truly on getting the essence (*rasa*), one becomes blissful. For who indeed could live, who breathe, if there were not this bliss in space? This verily is it that bestows bliss."[2] The altar of the diaphragm that rhythmically pumps the life-sustaining prāṇa is the basis for this joy. In meditative states, when the breath is made tranquil and serene, this joy arises again and again. Simply by breathing, we rejoice in prāṇa. For the yogi, the distilled and rarefied prāṇa, which is none other than consciousness (*citta*) itself, is a means to rejoice. This prāṇa is the source of citta, the intelligent wakefulness in the body. In the act of breathing, the *prāṇa-citta* is perpetually enlivened.

At the altar of the midchest, we aim to make the diaphragm free of restriction so that its movements are fluid and uninhibited; in this way, the very rhythm of the breath deepens in recurring cycles. When the intonations and cadence of the breath are smooth and rhythmic (intoning the classical mantra *Om* is conducive to this), we are *altered.* Nuanced changes take place in cardiovascular rhythm, brain function, and hormonal secretion, exalting the vibratory spirit.

As we have seen, it is impossible to separate the pulsating rhythms of the lungs, heart, and diaphragm. In fact, the heart rests directly on top of the diaphragm in such a way that its membranous covering, the pericardium, is continuous with the superior surface of the diaphragm. Every time we breathe our heart moves. When the duration of the breath is lengthened and the diaphragm becomes more supple, the heart is exercised and its muscular walls become more pliant. A heart that is more responsive is also more receptive to joy. Unfortunately most people's breath is shallow in measure (the average breath cycle being a mere three seconds), and constriction in the diaphragm weakens the biochemical fusion of spirit and flesh.

PRACTICE

The Altar of Devotion

This meditation uses creative visualization to access the sentiment of *bhakti* (devotion) within the respiratory rhythm. In this practice, the diaphragm is made sacrosanct while its motion is meant to generate feelings of deep acceptance.

Assume a comfortable seated position and as you breathe, sense the rise and fall of your diaphragm. Allow your breathing to be easy and fluid. Imagine your diaphragm to be a living altar and sense the way your heart suspends on top of this flowing altar. With each breath, feel the way your heart is lifted with the rhythmic motion of your diaphragm. Then visualize an image of a loved one, a divine being, a teacher, or an animal for whom you have unconditional love on top of the altar. Do this in the same way that you might place a photo or statue on an altar in your home or in a space devoted to practice. Let enter your heart someone who is a source of genuine vitality and kindness, someone who is a source of both nourishment and love. Observe the way this being helps to fill the space of your heart with gratitude. Allow your breath to be full of acceptance. Reflect on how the motion of each and every one of your breaths sustains this feeling of acceptance. Allow the entity on your altar to foster nonjudgmental awareness inside of you. Allow the goodwill of this being to pervade your entire chest and a feeling of spaciousness to fill your entire body. Notice how soft and supple your breath becomes as a result of this visualization. Remain for ten to twenty minutes. This meditation is helpful to heal from grief, loss, or despair.

Prāṇa, Nāḍīs, and the Pulse of Life

Prāṇa is likened to wind (*vāyu*), currents of living air that flow through and animate myriad channels (nāḍīs) in the subtle body. It is impossible to identify exactly the physical structures that correspond to the nāḍīs. Some say that nāḍīs, like Chinese meridians, are purely energetic and have no physiological counterparts. For teaching purposes, I imagine that the nāḍīs are vessels in the body that transport blood, lymph, and nerve impulses. The *Śiva Saṁhitā* states that 350,000 nāḍīs transport prāṇa—and consciousness—to every molecule in the body. The word *nāḍī* in Sanskrit evolves out of the root *nād,* meaning to move or flow. Nāḍīs pervade the body like infinitesimal veins. They are akin to fibril, feather-fine patterns in a leaf, water crystal, or sponge. Nāḍīs are interior rivulets that flow through all channels in the body from large vessels down to miniscule tubules.

The bioelectric prāṇa pulse circulates with the blood through arteriole channels and flows through nerve pathways that conduct impulses to all living tissues. Neurotransmitters cruise across synapses, spark sensory and motor neurons, and create a body electric.

The intricacy and complexity of the nervous system are phenomenal. Via yoga poses, the nāḍīs are alternately activated or pacified, opened or closed, in order to regulate the flow of prāṇa.

In yoga, prāṇa is not merely a biochemical force but is associated with spirit (in-*spira*-tion). In the Upanisads, prāṇa is sacrosanct and its amplifying force is referred to as *brahman*. The word *brahman* suggests the living breath (the name may have correlations with the name Abraham in the Old Testament), and thus when uttering the word *brahma*, the pronunciation of the sound *ah* invokes the Absolute. *Brahman* is synonymous with prāṇa; it is the beginning, middle, and end of all life. A verse in the *Taittirīya Upanisad* proclaims, "He knew that *prāṇa* is *brahman*. For truly beings here are born from *prāṇa*, when born they live by *prāṇa* and into *prāṇa*, when departing, they enter."[3]

Prāṇāyāma

It is remarkable that we can alter the inherent rhythm of the breath as it passes in and out of our lungs. Prāṇāyāma is our primary means of amplifying the prāṇa. We not only become the observer of our breath but the actor, commanding the breath by lengthening, quickening, or arresting it. In the physical disciplines of traditional yoga, prāṇāyāma is the means to enhance the presence of the divine, life-sustaining force.

In Latin, this force is called *anima*—the breath, the spirit, the soul, or vital force—which correlates with the Sanskrit verbal root *an*, meaning to breathe. The word *prāṇa* is built on this verbal root *an*, and prāṇāyāma, the regulation of the breath, is the central discipline of classical yoga. *Yama* is a word that suggests restraint and extension—that is, the breath can be held in check, sustained, emptied, or elevated. The word *prāṇāyāma* also implies a loosening or unfettering of the breath, if we translate the word as *prāṇa-ayama*. *Āyama* means unrestrained or unconfined, suggesting that ultimately the intention behind prāṇāyāma is not to confine the breath but to free it.

The word *yama* appears significantly in the Katha Upanisad where the deity Yama presides over the realm of the dead. In Hindu mythology, Yama is the ultimate restrainer. When the breath is fully restrained and the prāṇa can no longer move, life is exhausted. In this light, we could think of prāṇāyāma as the slow means to encounter death while living—a most difficult and perplexing task. In prāṇāyāma practice, this is accomplished by touching the very nadir of the breath at the end of the exhalation. In Sanskrit, the expiration phase of breathing is called the *rechaka*, literally the "exiting or emptying breath." Completely eliminating the breath is analogous to the supreme state of yogic meditation called *nirvāṇa*, which is a departure from the cycles of rebirth as suggested by early Buddhist teachings. Nirvāṇa literally means to "blow out," to extinguish, or simply to exhaust. One of the primary aims of yoga is to exhaust the confines of the limited, restricted self. In Patañjali's Yoga Sutras, this is accomplished namely by "exhausting the restless activity in the mind" (*citta vṛtti nirodhaḥ*). The act of exhausting the clatter of the mind is closely tied to exhalation, the dissolution phase of breathing.

The Paradox of Breathing and the Paradox of Mind

The movement of the entire rib basket with the diaphragm is not easy to grasp, for its motion is essentially paradoxical. For instance, when we imagine inhalation, we usually think of an upward expansion, yet the primary motion of the diaphragm during an in-breath is downward. And when we imagine exhalation, we have the impression of a downward movement, yet exhalation involves an upward pull of the diaphragm. This inverse dynamic, a kind of paradox regarding the upside-down breath, has interesting parallels with the nature of consciousness, especially as related to meditation and prāṇāyāma.

We must inquire, what is prāṇa and is it different from consciousness itself? Throughout all the meditative traditions, breathing lies at the heart of mindfulness training, so when we are discussing the breathing mechanism we are also referring to the mind. In yoga, it is said that breath (prāṇa) and mind (citta) are reciprocal. They travel together like two fish in a school. In the way that the mechanics of breathing are "upside down," consciousness is "inside out." This is due to the mind's capacity to perceive the things of the world while unable to perceive itself. It is like an eye that while looking outward does not see its own form. One of the chief aims of the yoga path is for consciousness to behold itself, and given the inverse operation of the thinking mind, this goal is extremely difficult to attain. The Tibetan Dzogchen meditation master Tulku Urgyen Rinpoche described awareness in this way: "Sentient beings are never apart from the unchanging, innate nature of mind for even an instant, yet they do not see it. Just as the nature of fire is heat and the nature of water is moisture, the nature of our mind is rigpa, non-dual awareness."[4]

"Seeing" this nondual awareness lies at the heart of all yoga training and involves a reversal of the inside-out attribute of everyday mind. In Zen meditation this reversal comes about by a backward movement, wonderfully described as "taking the backward step," or "turning the lantern of awareness back on itself."

For yogis, prāṇāyāma is the quintessential way to engage the paradoxical character of the mind. Prāṇāyāma helps to clarify the upside-down nature of the prāna-citta. While prāṇāyāma addresses breathing patterns, meditation serves to turn the "lantern of awareness" back on itself, revealing the "inside-out" nature of the mind. In yogic training, the quintessential way to accomplish this is by fusing or interpermeating mind and breath. When citta and prāṇa merge, the mind is able to see its nondual nature.

The interrelationship of breath and mind heralds back to some of the original teachings on yoga. In the Upanisads, prāṇa is the very essence of being. Prāṇa is vast and all pervasive, "smaller than the small, greater than the great" as suggested in the Kaṭha Upaniṣad. It is the life-force in a tumbleweed, the movement of the stars, and the heartbeat inside a fish. It is thought to be both the source of all physiological activity and the creative aspect of the world. While it is life itself, it is also the vast anonymous into which all things dissolve in the end.

The yoking together of mind and breath lies at the heart of all yogic training and is what sets the physio-spiritual discipline of yoga apart from other activities that use breath mechanics such as weight lifting, swimming, calisthenics, and Pilates. While these disciplines may require careful integration of the breath, they do not intend to yoke breathing and awareness together in such a way that the practitioner merges into a vast and ultimately unnameable plenum. In yoga, mindful, absorptive breathing enables the prāṇa-citta to experience itself as boundless. This is the state of undifferentiated awareness, the experience of oneness or samādhi. It is the end result of the magical alchemical infusion of prāṇa and citta.

PRACTICE

The River of Breath

An analogy I like to use to describe the indivisibility of mind and breath is that of a leaf (the mind) that has fallen into a river (the breath). When the mind suspends on the current of breath like a leaf bobbing in the current and when we follow our breath without distraction, a sense of deep calm prevails. This practice guides you through the experience of absorbing the mind into the current of the breath.

Begin by taking a comfortable seated position in such a way that you support your pelvis on a six-inch lift. Observe the steady flow of your breath. Allow the edges of your diaphragm to be supple. Enter the stream of your breath. Allow your breath to run continuously like a flowing current of water. Follow the stream of your breath and have faith in its course. It may meander here and there but always comes back to the fluid nature of breath. Don't push the river but allow it to be natural. As you settle into the meditation, visualize the river of your breath slowing down. Like the way a river deepens and widens when there is little grade, allow the murmur of your breath to become soft and unhurried.

Then imagine your mind is a leaf fallen into the stream of your breath. Allow your mind-leaf to suspend on the river of your breath and to bob, lift, and settle with the current. Wherever the current of your breath moves, so the leaf of your awareness follows. There should be no division between leaf and water, mind and breath. Notice how your leaf moves on inhalation and on exhalation. Sense the way your awareness drifts steadily on your breath. By the end of this meditation, observe the feeling of levity and calm in your mind. Stay for twenty minutes and afterward lie in śavāsana to release your spine.

In this chapter we have made it over the divide of the respiratory diaphragm, a significant crossing within the body. In so doing, we have passed from the dark depths of the subterranean gut en route to the more spacious realm of the heart, throat, and cranium. As we move into the structures superior to the diaphragm, the biorhythms of the body become all the more subtle. In our journey through the chakras to the top of the spine, we push beyond the edges of the physical and to the vibratory realm of spirit. We have seen in this chapter the metaphysical link between breathing, prāṇa, and consciousness. As we explore the upper chakras, we move further into more delicate strata of the subtle body. The glands, nerves, and sensory organs associated with the upper vertebral column are extremely sensitive. We will see, however, that the more refined and impressionable a structure, the more vulnerable it is to strain.

6

THE LUNGS AND THE LOTUS HEART

The Epicenter of Feeling

Waves rise
under a floating
lotus leaf.
My heart is moved
to touch you.

—Toshiyori Minamoto[1]

Contemplate to capacity
all the pain
of the human condition.

—Lama Mipham[2]

The lungs and heart are inseparable. An elaborate system of vessels spans the two organs so that if the heart were lifted from the chest cavity, as in cadaver studies, the lungs that are entwined with the heart would inevitably follow. The lungs and heart are not only structurally interwoven; as the body's primary repository for sentiment, together they filter emotion. The heart-lung chakra is heralded for being the epicenter of devotional feeling. This feeling, called *bhava* in Sanskrit, includes sentiment of tenderness and love. It is a state where empathy and kindness flourish, in part due to a genuine capacity to feel suffering, both personal suffering and the pain of all sentient beings. However, residues of emotional pain (*dukha*) confine the heart-lung and inhibit the subtle body.

In this chapter we investigate the anatomical structures of the lungs, pericardium, and heart, and review how the chest is the body's primary location for vibratory rhythms, pulses that can be felt through the entire body. We will explore the key role that the heart plays as the seat of the inner Seer in classical yoga. In yoga, the metaphorical heart is indivisible from consciousness, and thus a synthesis of heart and mind is critical for spiritual renewal and transformation.

Prenatal Lungs

What is it that initiates breathing? Is it simply muscular activity of the diaphragm, an involuntary reflex? The breath flows of its own accord, so one could live a lifetime and never have any regard for the breath. So what sets the lungs in motion?

In fetal development the lungs and entire pulmonary mechanism are latent, asleep like a hibernating fish. Barring connection to the outside air, the fetus need not generate its own oxygen, for it receives oxygenated blood from its mother via the placenta and umbilical cord. The moments after birth involve a radical shift for the lungs and diaphragm as they emerge from incubation, because, like a fish that has landed on shore, they are suddenly made to gape open and start pumping. At birth, the lung tissue and associated nerves spark open and the entire breathing mechanism kicks in. A smooth and rhythmic tempo of breath can take hours, days, or potentially a lifetime to coordinate. For many the first breath is traumatic. In a moment of life or death, the lungs gasp for air and the first neurological signal imparted to the lungs is often one of distress. The struggle to suck air in at birth may leave traces of strain and apprehension in the subtle body. Through years of breath-awareness training the respiratory rhythm may be reset—slowly, sensitively, and delicately—so that the shock waves triggered at birth may dissipate altogether.

PRACTICE

Sensing Your Breath Print

In this exercise the objective is to become aware of the inherent rhythm of your own breath and to identify with what my colleague Richard Rosen calls the "breath print." In the way that we each have unique thumbprints and fingerprints, we each have a unique respiratory rhythm. Prior to altering the breath in prāṇāyāma training, it is valuable to come to know your breath print.

Lie on your back and prop your spine six to twelve inches with folded blankets or a bolster. When you lie down, position the end of the bolster so that it supports your lower ribs at the level of your kidneys. Place a blanket or pad under your head so that your head does not tilt backward. Your forehead should be slightly higher than the bridge of your nose. Extend your legs out so that your feet are slightly wider than hip-width apart and rest your arms away from your trunk with your palms turned toward the sky.

Begin this prāṇāyāma preparation by softening your eyes and melting the skin of your face. Draw your ears inside so that you listen to the rhythm of your breath. Avoid manipulating or trying to engineer your breath at this initial stage. Release the weight of your spine into the prop and allow the weight of your arms and legs to sink into the floor. Be sure to let go of any peripheral holding in your limbs. Simply observe your breath's amplitude, depth, and rhythm. Notice your breath just as it is. This is your breath print. The following observations will help you gain sensitivity in your lungs: Observe how your breath brushes the back of your throat and filters down into your lungs. Observe the rise and fall of your belly as your breath moves in and out. Where does your breath make contact with your ribs? How does your breath flow into your back ribs, side ribs, and frontal ribs? Place your palms on top of your lower ribs and breathe into your palms. Notice the way your breath moves into your left hand and left lung. Notice the movement of your ribs under your right hand and into your right lung. Is there a difference in the motion and responsiveness of your right lung versus your left lung?

This information will help you determine which lung is more dominant. Remain for five to ten minutes, then roll off of the bolster to your right side prior to coming up to sitting.

The Hand-Lung Connection

In the motor development of an infant the crawling phase establishes foundational patterns for all movement. Bilateral development is essential for orienting the two sides of the body and promoting neurological advancement in the brain. Crawling initiates development within the lungs, hands, arms, shoulders, and the two domes of the diaphragm. Children who skip the cross-crawl phase may suffer from poor integration of their right and left sides. This may result in poor spatial awareness, lack of coordination, and compromised balance. Most practices of the internal arts—whether yoga, tai chi, Feldenkrais, or qigong—educate and integrate the body's two sides while orienting toward the body's midline.

In traditional Chinese medicine, the lung, pericardium, and heart meridians pass from the hand, through the arm, to the chest cavity. In the way that the tips of the toes are points of flow for the meridians within the leg, the fingertips conduct circulation of chi into the arms and trunk. Within the distal points of the hand, the thumb is the source of the lung meridian, the tip of the middle finger begins the pericardium meridian, and the little finger is the start of the heart meridian (fig. 6.1).

Kinetic forces traveling along the arm and hand directly stimulate circulation

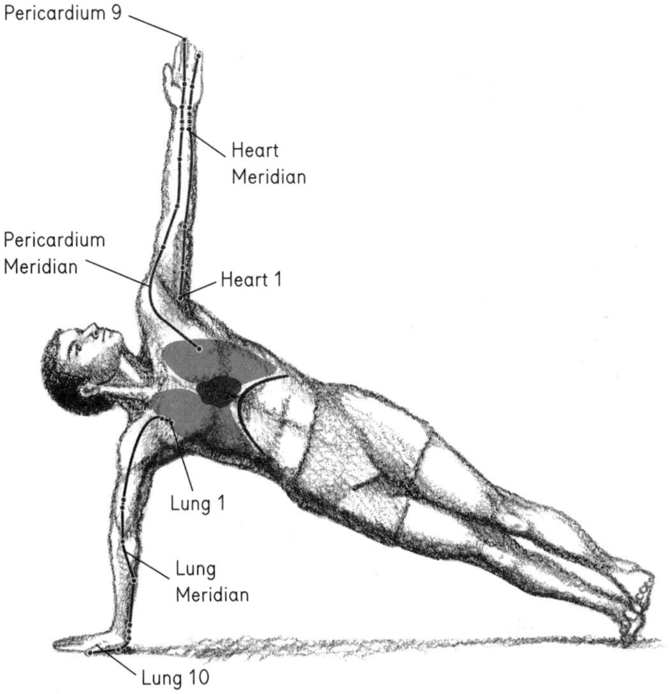
Pericardium 9
Heart
Meridian
Pericardium
Meridian
Heart 1
Lung 1
Lung
Meridian
Lung 10

Figure 6.1 Heart, Lung, and Pericardium Meridians in Vasiṣṭhāsana

through a large neurovascular bundle that transits under the collarbone and along the inside corridor of the arm called the thoracic outlet. This includes the vital structures that are the lifeline to the arm—the radial nerve, radial artery, and vein. In the way that we noted the "sacred seam" of the inside leg, the sacred seam of the arm is the thumb side of the arm. Postures that stretch and release the inside arms help improve the circulation of blood, lymph, and nerve. Positions like downward-facing dog pose, handstand, and *vasiṣṭhāsana* (side plank pose) stimulate movement through the heart, lung, and pericardium meridians. Thus, when students bear weight on their arms, it has immediate and powerful effects on increasing circulation into their lungs and heart.

PRACTICE

Opening the Sacred Seams of the Inside Arms

This sequence of poses promotes flow through the meridians and nāḍīs of the hand, while strengthening the muscles of the shoulder and chest cavity. It opens the lung tissues by stretching the meridians and blood vessels of the inside arms that pass from the arms to the chest.

Vasiṣṭhāsana

Begin in downward-facing dog pose. Actively divide your fingers and spread the bones of your hands. Place your right hand approximately four inches in front of your right shoulder as you pivot to the left. Align your right hand with the outer edge of your right foot. Stack your left leg on top of your right as you turn into vasiṣṭhāsana (side plank pose, named for the sage Vasiṣṭha). Activate your feet by pushing out through your heels, spreading your plantar fascia, and drawing your toes back toward your knees. Keep your legs firm. Press into the mat with the base of your index finger and thumb. The base of the thumb is a source point for the lung meridian (Lung 10), and pressing it down stimulates breath into the lung (see fig. 6.1). Actively radiate out through your fingers and draw upward through the center of your palm. Stretch the inside channel, the sacred seam, of your right arm while dynamically extending upward through your left arm. Feel the length and the span through all the connective tissues that orient along your inside forearms, upper arms, shoulders, and collarbones. Hold for fifteen to thirty seconds. To exit, pivot back to downward dog and then repeat on the other side.

The Arms as Gateways to the Lungs

ADHO MUKHA DAṆḌĀSANA

Begin on your hands and knees, set your shoulders directly over your wrists and your hips directly over your knees. Form a tepee with your hands by lifting up on the tips of your fingers. Then spread your fingers and the bones of your hands wide as you set your palms back down to the floor. This stretches the palm of the hand and the palmar fascia (akin to the plantar fascia of the foot) prior to weight bearing. Press the base of your index finger, the base of your little finger, and the outer and inner heels of each hand into the floor. These are the four corners of the hand, similar to the four corners of the feet discussed in chapter 1. Draw the center of each palm upward as you press the four corners down. This is the hand bandha or *hasta bandha*, a movement that resembles the lift of the center of the foot (pada bandha). Then lift your knees off the floor into *adho mukha daṇḍāsana.* The downward-facing staff pose is often mistakenly translated as plank pose, an important distinction, as the staff in yoga symbolically upholds the wisdom of the yoga lineage, whereas a plank is a run-of-the-mill slab of wood. Maintain your shoulders directly over your wrists and hold the outer edge of your arm bones firm. Draw your shoulder blades down your back away from the back of your skull. Continue to spread the platform of your hands wide. This will help expand your lungs, spread your ribs, and strengthen the intercostal muscles in your chest. Stay for thirty seconds to a minute then push back to downward dog or come down to rest in child's pose.

The Lung Tree

Our lungs resemble an upside-down tree, wherein the roots of the tree are located around the upper palate, the trunk is the windpipe (trachea), and the branches extend into the lobes of the lungs (fig. 6.2). Due to the amount of space that the heart occupies in the ventral chest cavity, the branches of the lung tree extend primarily to the back of the chest and down to the diaphragm. There are a multitude of twigs and branches, called bronchioles, that stem off the main trunks of the left and right bronchi. The bronchioles split again and again, terminating in superfine and porous membranous tips. These tips form clusters called alveoli, and approximately 300 million line each lung.

The exchange that occurs in breathing is somewhat like the process of photosynthesis. Throughout the alveoli, which resemble bunches of grapes, a gas-fluid exchange occurs by capillary action as oxygen-rich prāṇa is suffused into the bloodstream and carbon dioxide is drawn out of the blood. The extensive network of capillaries in the lung is so vast that if laid end to end they would travel a distance of one thousand miles.[3]

The aim of prāṇāyāma is to establish a full canopy for the lung tree. However, just as trees have withering tree branches that obstruct the flow of sap, nutrients, and water, it is common for some bronchioles to restrict the flow of air. Pleural clogs or adhesions are common, and may keep the air sacs from inflating, like leaf buds at the tips of tree branches that fail to open in spring. The cause of this may be due to lung diseases such as chronic obstructive pulmonary disease (COPD), emphysema, asthma, or chronic bronchitis. More commonly, stagnation in the lung is due to a previous lung infection, pneumonia, chronic coughing, smoking, physical trauma, or postural restrictions in and around the chest wall.

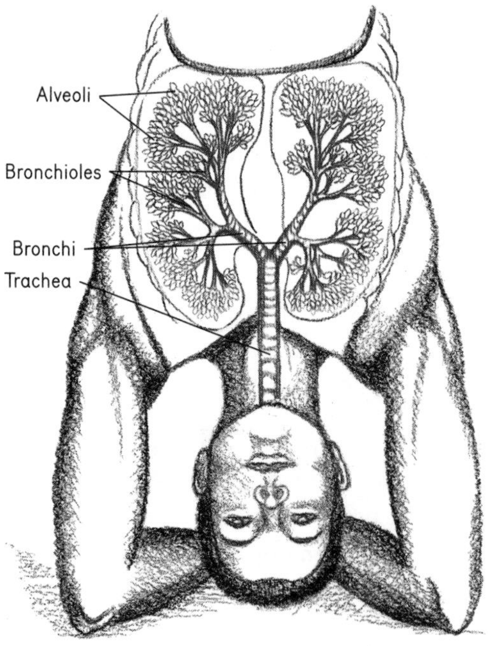

Figure 6.2 The Lung Tree in Śīrṣāsana

In an attempt to open their lungs, beginning prāṇāyāma students tend to overemphasize expansion of their ventral and superior chest, in part because the frontal chest is more visible. Over-emphasis on expanding the anterior chest compartment can potentially strain the heart. Avoiding such strain is the first principle in prāṇāyāma training, and for this reason, I encourage students to aim their breath into the outer canopy of the lungs at the side and back chest.

One of the best ways to foliate the lung tree is by inverting or partially inverting the body. Inversions such as headstand, shoulderstand, or supported bridge pose increase the circulation of blood and lymph through the lungs by changing the fluid pressure gradient between the abdominal cavity, diaphragm, and chest. Specifically, inversions benefit the lower lobes of the lungs that perch atop the respiratory diaphragm—in our lung tree this is the top of the pleural canopy. To exercise the lung tissue and facilitate full diaphragmatic breathing, backbends are also beneficial, especially backbends done with support of the thoracic spine.

PRACTICE

Supported Fish Pose

This exercise is valuable for people who spend considerable time at a keyboard, given the propensity for the shoulder girdle to drag forward when typing. Supported matsyāsana (fish pose) helps to actively spread the ribs, stretch the intercostal muscles, and open the anterior rib.

Prepare for the fish pose by placing a bolster or block underneath your shoulder blades. Set a folded blanket under the back of your head. Arch back over the block so that you trap both shoulder blades, pinning them against your back ribs. Be sure the block is positioned in such a way that it is directly under your shoulder blades and catches their lower margin (the inferior angle). Your head will extend back, and your neck will have a gentle arch. If you experience neck compression, elevate your head more.

The block should act as a fulcrum, lifting and spreading your ribs, collarbones, and sternum. Allow the weight of your shoulders to sink into the prop. Extend your arms out to the sides and then stretch your arms directly over your head and toward the floor. Stay in this pose for two to three minutes before pushing your elbows into the floor in order to come straight up to sitting.

Watering the Roots of the Lungs

When teaching breathing in prāṇāyāma training, I like to use the image of watering a tree. In the way that a gardener should soak a tree down to its roots, it is important to irrigate the lungs with oxygen during mindful breathing. In full diaphragmatic breathing, it is advisable to guide the breath deep into the lobes of the lungs.

Without articulating the breath into the lower lungs, students are inclined to quickly "pop" or force the breath into the upper lobes. A high, clavicular breath can potentially cause strain in the neck and heart, trigger excitation, and cause agitation. Some yoga practices overemphasize a quick pumping breath like the breath of fire. While stimulating, this rapid succession of breath fails to irrigate the deeper lung tissue and can lead to ungrounded psychological states. When the breath infuses the lower lung tissue, it promotes a sense of serenity and calm, building *sthira* and *sukha* within the breath—stability and ease.

Figure 6.3 Topography of Lungs: The Lung Lobes and the Five Elements

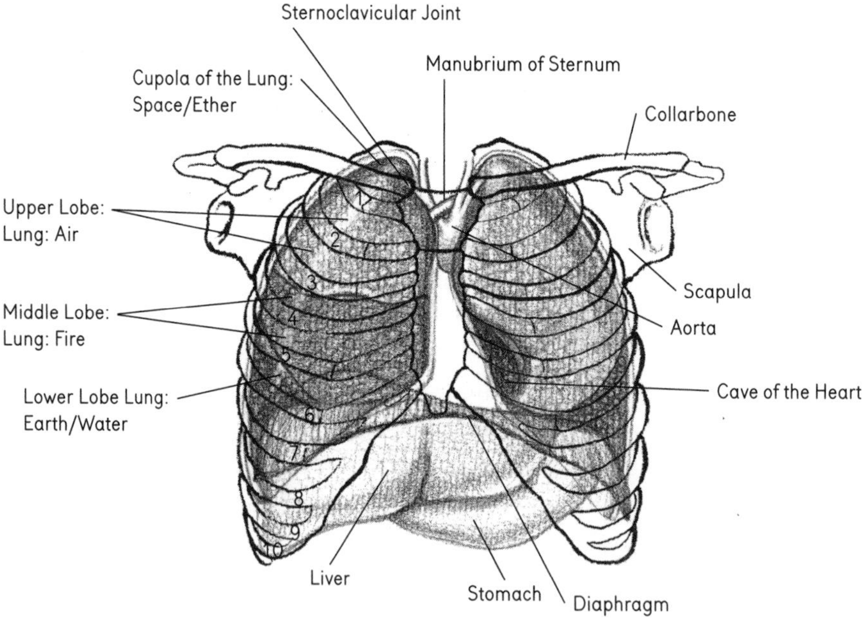

AN ELEMENTAL MAP OF THE BODY

If we map the four primary elements—earth, water, fire, and air—schematically onto the lung, we identify the lower lobes as earth and water, the middle lobes as fire, and the upper lobes as air. Since the earth element is associated with the inferior lung, guiding the breath into the lower lobe helps to settle and deepen respiratory rhythm. Simply breathing into the middle and upper lung increases fire and wind and can result in restlessness, busyness, and anxiety. Panicky and agitated feelings may cause the breath to flutter in the upper lungs. When students soften and elongate their breath (as in the "Sensing Your Breath Print" exercise earlier in this chapter) and guide it into the lung basin, they benefit from the more stabilizing and grounding effects of the earth and water elements (fig. 6.3).

PRACTICE

Ventilating the Lungs with Viparīta Daṇḍāsana

In this posture, you will dramatically open your upper chest cavity and expand your lungs. It is important to warm up with preparatory poses prior to performing this position. Start your practice session by doing a series of twists to release your spine. Then do preparatory backbends in order to generate extension in your lower back, such as cobra pose, upward-facing dog pose, bridge pose, and *ustrāsana* (camel pose), holding each pose for 30 seconds to a minute.

For *viparīta daṇḍāsana* (inverted staff pose) you will need a folding chair (preferably one without a backrest), blanket, strap, and two blocks. Start by sitting backward through the chair on a folded blanket with your feet on the floor. Loop the strap over your upper thighbones so that your feet are hip-width apart. Hold the top of the chair with your hands and arch backward, hooking the base of your shoulder blades on the front edge of the chair. Be sure that your shoulder blades do not slide off the lip of the seat. Pull your hands against the back bar to actively spread and open your lungs, collarbones, and ribs. Should you get back pain, remain with your knees bent.

Set a block or other support under your head so that there is no strain on your neck. Then slide your arms back along the inner edge of the chair and clasp the back legs. Pull with your hands in order to spread your upper chest. Breathe normally and observe the

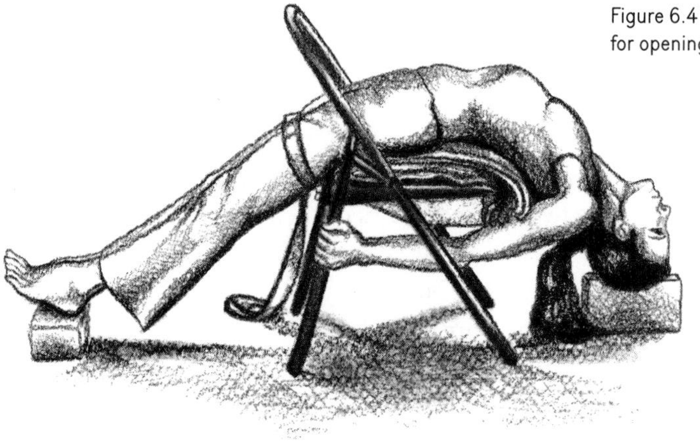

Figure 6.4 Viparīta Daṇḍāsana for opening the Lung-Heart

stretch of your iliopsoas muscles, diaphragm, and lungs. To elongate your spine further, extend your legs (fig. 6.4). If by extending your legs you experience back pain, then either set your feet higher by placing them on a block or bend your knees. Stay for two to four minutes.

To come out, bend your knees, release your hands, and once again clasp the back of the chair. Plant your feet firmly and pull with your hands so that you exit straight upward without twisting or torquing your spine. Once upright sit facing backward in the chair for a minute and feel the expansion of your upper chest and lungs.

The Crown of the Lung

If you slide your fingers into the indented space immediately above your clavicle, you are palpating the tissues around the uppermost dome of the lung called the cupola (fig. 6.3). In architecture, a cupola, shaped like an overturned cup, is constructed atop a building. It is a design that enables more light and air to enter. In the architecture of the upper torso, if we imagine the collarbones to be the roofline of the torso, then the cupolas of the lungs that jut above the collarbones provide a feeling of upward expansion. In our map of the elements associated with the lungs, the coronet of the uppermost lung is homologous to the atmospheric elements, air, and space/ether (see fig. 6.3). When the breath ascends to the cupola of the lung, during relaxed and open breathing, feelings of levity and joy result.

When the crown of the lung becomes light and spacious, a sentiment of bliss is palpable in the subtle body. However, in the face of threat the breath can become trapped in the stratosphere of the top lung. If caught in a startle response, the upper chest can heave and tense. Shock, panic, or fear can lead to feelings of constriction and shortage of breath. In the face of trauma, the top lung may constrict and the area around the collarbones—including the delicate muscles of the throat—are adversely affected. In reference to the feeling of terror, we have the expression in English, "My heart was in my throat." However, it may be more appropriate given the location of the cupola of the lung to say, "My lungs were in my throat."

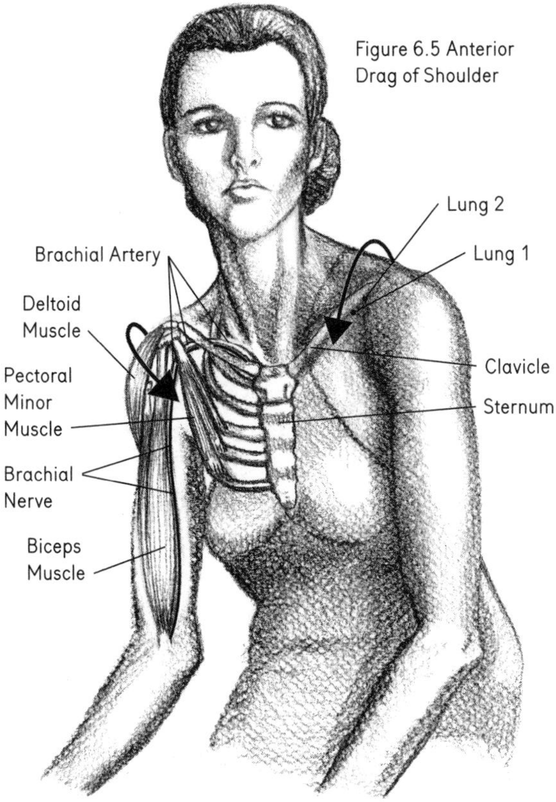

Figure 6.5 Anterior Drag of Shoulder

Near the thoracic outlet at the lateral edge of the collarbones are the primary points for the lung meridian in traditional Chinese medicine. Just inferior to the outermost collarbone, in the small indentation known as the clavipectoral fascia, are the acupressure landmarks for Lung 1 and 2 points (figs. 6.1 and 6.5). These points are needled to help relieve colds, asthmatic conditions, difficulty in breathing, and pulmonary disorders. In postural dynamics, it is common for the shoulders to curl forward such that the shoulder, upper arm (humerus), and chest converge, narrowing and compressing the first two points of the lung channel. This is often due to foreshortening of the biceps, anterior deltoid, pectoralis major, and pectoralis minor muscles. This forward curl of the shoulder complex is a common cause of shoulder dysfunction.

Yoga positions that best relieve congestion in the upper chest and thoracic outlet are shoulderstand and *halāsana* (plow pose). Initially these poses may cause compression due to predisposed strain and tension at the anterior shoulder. For this very reason, students often have an aversion to these inverted poses. However, when done correctly (I teach both plow and shoulderstand using the support of a bolster, chair, wall, or blankets), there should be very little pressure on the neck. When plow and shoulderstand are done correctly, blood and lymph irrigate into the upper torso, thereby opening the region near the first two acupressure points of the lung. When the upper torso is bathed in blood and lymph, there is a chance for greater levity in an area of the body that is prone to congestion and tension. This lift is difficult to achieve due to the way people carry physical, psychological, and emotional burdens in their shoulders.

PRACTICE

A Bridge to Shoulderstand

This position provides lightness and space to the uppermost chest while facilitating the flow of blood and lymph back to the heart.

Begin by setting up a three- to six-inch-high blanket pad for your shoulders. Lie on your back so that your shoulders are at the edge of the blankets and your head is on the floor. Position a chair so that it is right up to your blanket platform. Hold the front legs of the chair with your hands as you place your feet on the seat of the chair. Then pull with your hands, press your feet into the chair seat at its front edge, and lift your pelvis off the floor. Be sure to tuck your outer shoulders underneath you, as if you are tucking a fitted sheet under the corner of a mattress. Lift your pelvis as far upward as possible by pulling the legs of the chair with your hands. Stay for two minutes, then come down to rest in such a way that you place your calves onto the chair and your pelvis on the blankets.

The Impressionable Lungs

The yoga heart is celebrated for being the epicenter of feeling in the body, and while this is true, we must take into account the highly responsive and sensitive makeup of the lungs. Lung tissue is extremely light and fragile due to the fact that the capillary membranes at the outermost tips of the bronchioles (the alveoli and alveolar sacs) must be fine enough to permit gas absorption into the bloodstream.

A disarticulated lung reveals how vulnerable the lungs are and how susceptible they are to disfigurement. The tender and spongy lung tissue can easily wither, blotch, and become constricted. The lungs are vulnerable to defacement from smoke, airborne particulates (either material or chemical), pollen, or pollutants.

The lungs are entirely receptive as they filter and absorb oxygen from incoming air. Structurally, the lungs are impressionable, meaning delicate and pliable. The tissue of a healthy lung is gelatinous; it is possible to insert a finger up to the first knuckle into a living lung. The lungs are continuously exposed to the outside environment, given the constant exchange with the outside air. Not only do the lungs absorb air; they are also vulnerable to the atmospheric whims of mood and sentiment.

The lungs are also impressionable in an emotional sense. Below the radar of cognition, the lungs are susceptible to a whole spectrum of feeling states ranging from the slightest sentiment to an overwhelming, strong feeling. Feelings, especially grief and sadness, imprint onto the lung tissue. The impressionable lung is most evident in a young child. Disposed to strong feelings, the child self-regulates by laughing, crying, or screaming. Unfortunately adults withhold emotion such as fear, grief, and anger, and the lungs do not exorcise strain. Thus, when healing the subtle body, it is important to not only filter the lungs through āsana and prāṇāyāma but process the many complex feelings that absorb into the lung tissue.

The Lungs and Depression

It is interesting to note that in traditional Chinese medicine the lungs are considered the seat of grief in the body while the heart is the abode of joy. The bittersweet blend of sorrow and joy is inherent to the human experience. Grief takes root in the lungs and when it festers, melancholy and sadness prevail. Depression inevitably involves the lungs, due to the way the lungs activate prāṇa, and prāṇa is correlated with spirit. During episodes of depression, the lungs tend to shut down, muting the flow of prāṇa.

When depression sets in, it shrouds the lungs. In some cases, people who are depressed smoke cigarettes in an attempt to pry the lung tissue open, yet the expansive effects are merely temporary. Yogāsana and prāṇāyāma are beneficial to help counter depression, because they foster sustained opening of the lungs.

Depression, whether it has a genetic component or is linked to an experience of great loss in the course of a lifetime, involves biochemical changes too complex to detail here. Yet the lungs are our lifeline, they are our point of contact with the world at large, and the intake of oxygen-rich air has immediate and far-reaching effects on our nervous system. Because the lungs are vessels bearing and distributing the vital prāṇa, they are inevitably involved in deep-seated states of mood and emotion.

If breathing could be compared to tidal flow, then inhalation is the incoming tide and exhalation is the outgoing tide. Both are necessary for rhythmic and dynamic respiratory flow. Generally speaking, we prescribe backbends for people who suffer from depression. Backbends invite the ribs, intercostals, sternum, clavicles, and the heart-lung tissue to expand (fig. 6.4). Like the incoming tide, backbends increase the capacity for inhalation as prāṇa rushes into the lungs. Forward bends, however, support and complement the exhalation phase of the breath and help to quiet and subdue pranic rhythms.

For people who suffer from depression, we recommend prāṇāyāma practices that focus on inhalation in order to stretch and open the lung tissue. *Viloma prāṇāyāma* (against-the-grain breath) allows the inhalation to swell via small waves. In this breath, we build the amplitude of the inhalation by inserting short pauses as the breath mounts—that is, inhale pause, inhale pause, inhale pause. This breath generates pliability and resiliency in the rib basket in order to accommodate greater breath volumes. For depression, a synchronous breathing pattern where the duration of the inhalation and exhalation are of the same length, called *samavṛtti prāṇāyāma* (equal-ratio breath), is helpful to regulate respiratory, hormonal, and neurological activity.

PRACTICE

Equalizing the Flow of Breath (Equal-Ratio Breath)

In this prāṇāyāma, the inhalation and exhalation are even in length. This breath builds greater equilibrium in the respiratory rhythm while generating greater equanimity in the emotional body.

Assume a comfortable seated posture on a four- to six-inch support. Raise the top corners of your chest, countering any anterior drag of your shoulder. Be sure that your collarbones and upper chest spread wide and the region around your Lung 1 and 2 acupressure points are open (fig. 6.5). Begin with a slow soft breath, equalizing the length of both inhalation and exhalation. Be sure to find a ratio—say, a four-second inhale and a four-second exhale—that is appropriate for you and does not cause strain. In time you may extend the duration to as much as a seven-second inhale and seven-second exhale. After you have done the counting breath for five minutes, sit quietly with normal breath before lying down to rest.

PRACTICE

Interrupted Breath, Viloma I Prāṇāyāma (Against-the-Grain Breath)

This practice will help you develop greater range and responsiveness during inhalation.

Lie down onto the support of a bolster such that the bolster supports your spine from your head to your dorsal hinge (T12). Be sure to elevate your head with a folded blanket. Take time to prepare your body by following the instructions for "Sensing Your Breath Print" on page 162. Once you have reached a state of relaxed alertness and contacted the inherent rhythm of your breath, begin by exhaling deeply a few times in the way that an outgoing tide pulls away from shore. Now draw your breath approximately halfway into your chest and retain it for three to five seconds. Exhale slowly and empty your lungs. Avoid tensing or straining your muscles in any way. Repeat a few rounds of drawing your breath in, filling your lungs to 50 to 60 percent capacity, retaining for a short period, and exhaling.

Next, draw in your breath and fill approximately 50 percent of your lung capacity and pause. Then draw in another 20 to 25 percent and pause briefly again, before exhaling. Repeat this four to six times. Now draw your breath in to fill approximately 40 percent of your lung capacity and pause; draw in to 60 percent and pause; and then to 80 percent and pause. After exhaling, take several normal breaths. Be sure not to clench anywhere in your body. Don't be greedy; avoid the temptation to fill your lungs to the maximum. In this training, more is not necessarily better. Over time you can adjust the pauses and the length of the mini-retentions. Practice until the pauses for the interrupted breath are spontaneous and meet the needs of your lung capacity at any given time. Afterward, allow your breath to return to normal as you rest in śavāsana.

The Thoracic Outlet

The region of the upper thoracic cavity is a heavily trafficked area for both blood and nerve, like a tangle of major interstates that converge in a sprawling city. A considerable volume of blood flows through the region of the top chest at the base of the neck near the collarbones (see fig. 6.7). On the inside border of the sternum, blood surges out of the left side of the heart into the ascending aorta. Sizable bypasses exit off the aorta and travel into the cranium (carotid artery), into the dome of the uppermost chest, and out to the arms via the brachial artery (whose route begins at the subclavian artery). If you place your hand on the top notch of your sternum, you hover atop the snarl of nerve and blood traffic that passes through the upper thoracic cavity. Due to ventral drag of the shoulder (see fig. 6.5) and the effects of the red-light reflex discussed in the last chapter, the flow of blood and nerve in the upper thorax may be compromised.

Given that the rib basket is shaped like a cone—wide at the base along the rib angle and floating rib, and narrow at the top near the collarbones—it is easy for the thoracic outlet to become a bottleneck. At the top of the rib cone, the diameter of the first rib is remarkably narrow. If you create an oval with the pads of your thumbs and index fingers you form the approximate circumference of the first rib at the very top of the trunk. The collarbones attach to the sternum at the stout sternoclavicular joint; this is the only place where the entire shoulder complex and scapulae attach to the main part of the skeleton (see fig. 6.3).

The downward pull of the chest cavity can cause the sternum to topple and slip downward, constricting the accordion-like action of the ribs, intercostal muscles, and sternocostal joints. On the interior border of the sternum, there is a beautiful muscle shaped like a butterfly, called the transversus thoracis muscle. This muscle spans from the sternum to Ribs 2–6 on the inside surface of the frontal chest. In all poses, whether forward or backward bends, twists, or inversions, this muscle should remain wide. When there is ventral drag of the shoulder, the sternum, the transversus thoracis muscle, and the clavicles displace downward, retarding the circulation of blood through the upper chest, neck, head, and arms.

Sailing the Kite of the Sternum

Just as a kite suspends on atmospheric wind currents, so the sternum and heart float upward on the internal winds of breath. Anatomically the heart is attached to the posterior border of the sternum, so that whenever the sternum moves, the heart follows. Poses that actively stretch the sternum, such as taking the arms behind the back and clasping the fingers together, serve to lift and spread the kite sternum. Accompanied by full diaphragmatic breathing, we can imagine the sternum broadening widthwise like the horizontal axis through a kite, and extending lengthwise, like the vertical axis. In the way that a kite in the sky must be kept aloft at all times, in yoga practice, and particularly in seated meditation, one must sustain the lift of the sternal kite. During prāṇāyāma,

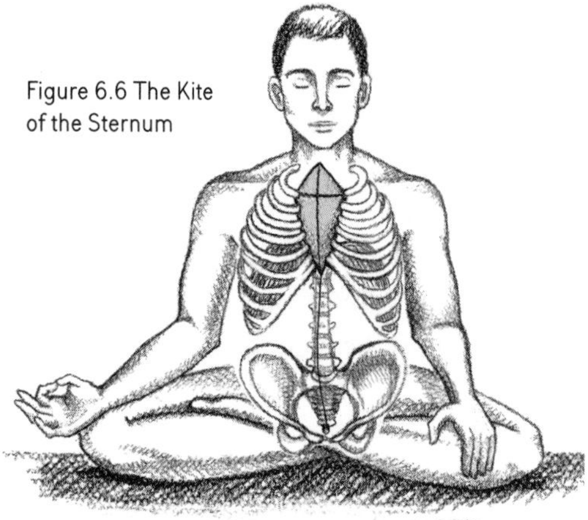

Figure 6.6 The Kite of the Sternum

when the chest cavity is inflated, the movements of the kite are constantly changing relative to the currents of prāṇa flowing in the chest. We can visualize the kite string of the sternum traveling through the diaphragm, back along the front margin of the spine, and down to the tailbone where the string is tethered. The tailbone serves to anchor and guide the kite to greater buoyancy via the action of mūla bandha (fig. 6.6). ◈

The First Two Ribs

Along with the sternum, the position of the collarbone and first two ribs is instrumental in maintaining breadth and openness in the lanes of arterial flow that transit through the upper thorax. My Rolfing instructor, Jan Sultan, taught that the placement of Ribs 1 and 2 is most critical for maintaining appropriate balance and integration of the arms, neck, and head. These first two ribs are directly below the clavicles in the upper chest (see fig. 6.3). Given the anterior pull of the shoulder girdle, the collarbones, together with Ribs 1 and 2, depress. Thus, when we stand in tāḍāsana, practice śīrṣāsana, or sit meditation, it is valuable to lift the first and second ribs and "float" the collarbones. I like to imagine slender balloons the width of pencils nestled below each collarbone enabling them to float.

The Eyes of the Heart

B. K. S. Iyengar once called the edges of the thoracic diaphragm just below the outer collarbones "the eyes of the heart." The eyes of the heart are in the same vicinity as the first two points of the lung meridian that were mentioned earlier. For optimal flow through the thoracic outlet, it is critical to keep the top upper portion of the chest free of constriction. Corollary to this anatomical reference, the eyes of the heart have a mystical sensibility that involves an inner Seer that sees without looking.

The eyes of the heart are apertures leading to metaphysical or spiritual connection. In the way that the third eye within the cranium has intuitive insight, the yoga heart has an uncanny capacity to see the invisible. "The heart is the organ with which one is able to see what is denied to the physical eye," wrote Jan Gonda in *The Vision of the Vedic Poets*.[4] The heart as seer or interior witness harkens back to the Upaniṣadic notion that there is a divine, omniscient being that dwells in everyone's heart. This being, called the *puruṣa,* resides within the heart as an all-pervading consciousness, entirely unaffected by the senses, cognition, or intellect:

> The *puruṣa*, the size of a thumb, the innermost self (*ātmā*),
> Always abides in the heart. One should steadfastly draw him
> out of the body,
> Like a reed from a sheath of grass.
> One should know him as bright and immortal
> One should know him as bright and immortal.[5]

This passage at the end of the *Kaṭha Upaniṣad* describes a delicate yoking of the innermost self. The image of extracting a reed steadily from its sheath speaks to a subtle unveiling within the heart and revelation of an inmost spirit—the *puruṣa*. It is a process that involves deftness and exquisite attunement to that which inevitably, and necessarily, eludes our normal perceptual capacity.

Opening the delicate realm of the heart, like drawing an interior stem from a grass sheath, requires tactful precision and only the slightest degree of force. In mature stages of practice within the internal arts we learn to apply a "forceless force" or an "effortless effort" in order to yoke the innermost self. The inner Seer is not something that can be conjured or deliberately called forth. The exquisite sensitivity of the heart requires the most refined attention and tender approach, one imbued with the qualities of metta (loving-kindness), patience, and nongrasping.

PRACTICE

Opening the Collarbones and the Eyes of the Heart

This practice lifts and expands the structures at the top outer corners of the chest in order to open the "eyes of the heart." Stand in tāḍāsana with a strap ready in one hand. Adjust the strap so that the circumference is just the width of your shoulders. Take your arms behind you, loop the strap around both arms, setting it just above your elbows. Then place your hands on your sacrum at the base of your spine. The strap should now be like a sling, holding your elbows in place so they cannot splay outward. Should your arms feel excessively restricted, loosen the strap. Those with more range of motion in the shoulders may tighten the strap so the loop is narrower than shoulder width. Now extend your arms toward the wall behind you with your palms facing each other. Raise your arms upward toward the ceiling; *be sure to keep your sternum lifted* so it does not collapse downward. This will reverse the tendency for the anterior shoulder to be pulled forward and down. Observe the lateral spreading of your collarbones, sternum, transversus thoracis muscle, and first two ribs. Fill your breath into your upper outer chest, thereby opening the eyes of the heart. Stay for two minutes.

Once you take the strap off, stand in tāḍāsana with your eyes closed for thirty seconds and use your inhalation to lift and spread the top of your chest. Feel levity and space below your collarbones, thereby widening the mystical eyes of your heart.

Protecting the Emperor of the Heart

In the midchest, immediately behind the breastbone, the right and left lung sandwich the heart and secure it firmly in place. The space in which the heart resides, between the fleshy overlapping lungs, is referred to as the cave of the heart (*hṛdaya guhā*). In the esoteric yoga tradition, this cave is home to the soul or innermost Seer.

Anatomically a protective covering, the pericardium, enshrouds the heart like a cocoon and secures it firmly to the top of the diaphragm. The excursion of the heart on the tidal rhythms of the breath is limited, for the pericardium adheres to the central tendon of the diaphragm. As we saw in chapter 5, the central tendon of the diaphragm moves very little while the borders of the diaphragm are mobile. Nevertheless, with every breath we take, the heart floats up and down like a tethered buoy inside a protected bay.

The protective stocking of the pericardium stabilizes the heart in the same way that the pleural membrane secures the lungs and the dura surrounds and protects the spinal cord. In traditional Chinese medicine, the pericardium is considered an organ and is thought to shelter the heart in the way that perimeter palace walls safeguarded the emperor in ancient China. In this sense, the pericardium protects the *shen,* or spirit that resides in the heart, and shields it from what traditional Chinese medicine identifies as "external pernicious influences." Not only is the pericardium a stabilizing physical sheath but it could be thought of as an energetic shield encasing the fragile, highly sensitive, and emotive heart.

In contemporary terminology the concept of pernicious influences, threatening forces that may invade the emperor's domain, suggests the assaultive effects of emotional trauma that can cause the psychospiritual sheathing around the heart to rupture. Emotional trauma in our culture is extensive, from the threat of a terrorist attack to the aftermath of shootings in public schools to the annihilation results of natural disasters. The effects of such trauma on the autonomic nervous system and the subtle body are all the more insidious because they may be invisible to the naked eye. War, violence, physical, sexual, and emotional abuse, environmental catastrophe, and the loss of a loved one are causes for profound fear, grief, anxiety, and feelings of isolation. When the energetic buffer around the heart is torn, especially in young

Figure 6.7
The Cave of the Heart

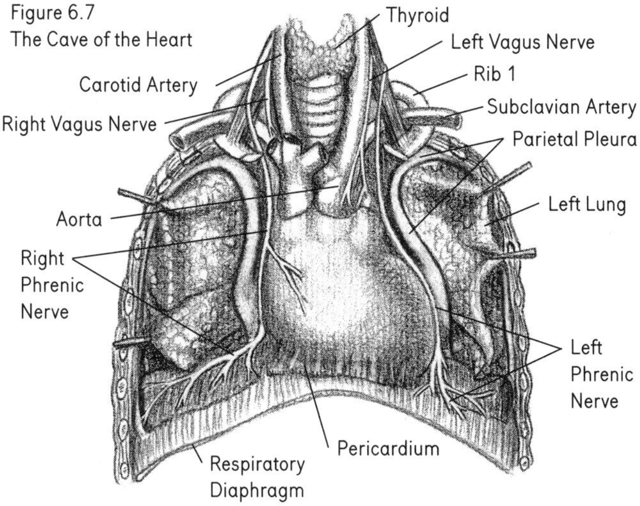

children, the spirit is left unguarded, and feelings of hurt, shame, and fear metastasize through the body. For this reason, traditional Chinese medicine treats the pericardium in cases of "sudden heart pain, palpitations, oppression of the chest, apprehension, propensity to fright, epilepsy, mania, agitation and restlessness . . . manic raving as if seeing ghosts or sudden fright disorder in children."[6]

PRACTICE

Mātaṅgi Mudrā and the Pericardium

In this exercise, we will practice *mātaṅgi mudrā*, which in Indian Tantra is one of the ten *mahāvidyas* (manifestations of the Divine Mother). This hand mudrā brings vitality and a dynamic lift to the chest (fig. 6.8). It is thought to enhance respiration and is best linked to the expansive phase of the inhalation. In meridian theory, the pericardium channel on each side of the body flows from the middle chest above the nipple (Pericardium 1) along the central axis of the arm to the tip of the middle finger (Pericardium 9). Thus, movements that activate the "middle ray" of the hand (the middle finger) actively tone and stretch the pericardial sinew channel (see fig. 6.1).

Sit comfortably on a four- to six-inch platform so that your spine is lifted and your shoulder blades recede down your back. Bring awareness to the rhythm of your breath and notice the energetic space around your heart. Visualize the pericardial sheathing that wraps your heart in a cocoon. What is the quality of sensation like in the energetic and physical membrane that enshrouds your heart? Does it feel thick, tight, or quivery? Does it feel fragile, constricted, or expansive? Reflect on any recent or distant circumstances in your life that may affect the shape, consistency, and tension of the pericardium.

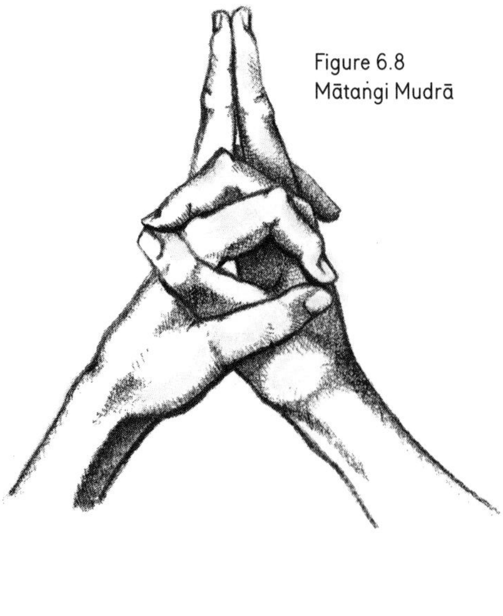

Figure 6.8
Mātaṅgi Mudrā

Take your hands in front of your chest in the prayer position, called *añjali mudrā*. Then interlace your fingers as if you are going to do śirṣāsana (headstand); this integrates the two brain hemispheres. Now extend your two middle fingers vertically and form two intersecting rings with the index finger and thumb of each hand. This is mātaṅgi mudrā. Be sure that the middle fingers are aligned symmetrically. Lightly press the center of your middle finger pads together. This stimulates the Pericardium 9, the jing well point of the pericardium meridian, used in TCM to reduce agitation in the heart plexus. Orient your middle fingers with the midline of your body along the central axis of the subtle body (suṣhumnā). Raise your elbows and broaden and lift your side ribs. Focus on the way your inhalation expands outward to your side ribs, back ribs, and front ribs. Remain for one to five minutes while sensing the strength and equanimity of the mudrā.

The Heart and Blood Pressure

Blood pressure changes constantly throughout the course of a day. Its rhythmic patterns are influenced by a multitude of factors including diet, time of day, activity level, hormonal regulation, and state of mind. Through attentive practice students of the internal arts can learn to track the oscillating patterns in their blood pressure. Some poses make the blood pressure rise (warrior poses and handstand, for example), and some lower blood pressure (such as seated forward bends and supported shoulderstand). It is useful to observe your blood pressure not only on the mat but also in the midst of everyday circumstances. When you are exerting yourself or you're under stress, your blood pressure will increase; when you are at rest, it will slow down. It is valuable to take your pulse by sensing the ongoing shifts in blood pressure. In this way you can begin to track states of inner activation that can have dramatic effects on the subtle body.

If the body systemically locks up and is rife with tension, the entire network of arteries and veins that carry blood in and out of the extremities may become compromised, impeding circulation. It is not only the pericardial sheathing and cardiac muscle tissue that restrict; the road map of arteries through the body may become sclerotic or fibrotic. When the arteries and veins do not readily expand and contract (spanda), the heart has to exert more in order to circulate the blood. When the vessel walls are pliable, they facilitate circulatory rhythm, performing like microhearts throughout the body.

When we do āsana, the circulatory pathways do not remain static. Stretching the myofascial layers of the body not only lengthens the musculature but also helps make the arteries and veins more tensile. The heart's capacity for local circulatory pressure is due to a dynamic balance between cardiac rhythm and the pump of the microvessels in the periphery. The most effective way to reduce blood pressure systemically is to make the cadence and tempo of the breath prolonged, slow, and featherlike. When there is less tension on the heart and on the arteries that carry blood out of the heart, the blood pressure drops. Reduced blood pressure is a prerequisite for states of internal meditation that heal the subtle body. When the body settles into a deep calm called *śamatā*, a synchronistic rhythm sets in involving the pericardium, heart, lung, diaphragm, and peripheral vessels. This quiescence not only has profound physiological effects on the body but also supports psychic absorption (samādhi) into the interior.

PRACTICE

Metta and Sensing Heart Rate

In order to reduce blood pressure, expand the prāṇa vāyu, and yoke the subtle body, it is valuable to promote states of empathetic awareness. This heart-centering meditation fosters deep relaxaton while prompting tender feelings of self-acceptance. By slowing the rythms of the heart, this practice induces calm and lowers blood pressure.

Sit comfortably and with clarity and gentleness bring awareness to the rise and fall of your breath. Feel any nuance of sensation around your diaphragm and heart. Observe the ways in which your breath pattern changes over time. As you follow your breath "frame by frame," cultivate a soft, steady cadence of breath.

Now listen for the beat of your heart in the left side of your chest cavity. Simply observing your heartbeat will connect you to the heart's subtle vibrations and promote feelings of empathetic awareness. Soak your awareness into your heartbeat the way rainwater soaks the ground after a storm. Notice the quality of feeling in your heart. Does your heart feel vacuous or full, weighty or light, guarded or open? Then evoke feelings of tenderness and receptivity in your heart. Allow your heart to be imbued with metta, or loving-kindness. Direct kindness toward yourself, making the following supplication: may I be free from physical pain, may I be free from psychological holding, may I be free from emotional suffering, and may I be spiritually awake. As you set this intention (*saṅkalpa*) notice any biochemical shifts that occur in your body. Once you tap the spirit of metta, or "all-pervading compassion," allow the feeling to spread throughout your chest. Observe not only your heart rate but any changes that take place in the micropulses throughout your wrists, hands, neck, and head. What changes can you detect? Bask in the warmth of this aspiration for ten to fifteen minutes. Afterward, lie down to rest.

The Phrenic Nerve and the Heart-Head Connection

The breathing mechanism is regulated by a bundle of neurons in the respiratory center of the brain. The action potential of this center is so powerful that even if peripheral nerves are severed, the mechanism that instigates breathing deep in the brain stem will continue for some time. Breathing is also activated by stretch receptors within the lung. These stretch receptors are strewn throughout the bronchioles and bronchi and refer back to the vagus nerve. Yet the primary nerve that innervates the diaphragm is called the phrenic nerve—a long, threadlike nerve that originates in the neck, descends along the heart, and ties onto the convex dome of the superior diaphragm (see fig. 6.7). The phrenic nerve has sensorimotor associations with the diaphragm and also has fibers that innervate the lungs and pericardium. The word *phrenic* is one of the few terms to suggest a direct correlation between breathing, heart, and mind (the Greek *phreno* connotes both mind and diaphragm).

The mind-breath or mind-heart affinity is celebrated in numerous passages throughout the earliest descriptions of yoga. Perhaps the best known is a verse that appears at the end of the *Katha Upaniṣad*, a passage that describes the merging of the individual self into absolute consciousness, *brāhman*. A profound physio-spiritual consummation, depicted archaically in the *Kaṭha Upaniṣad* as the state of immortality, involves a kind of bioelectric interfusion of heart and head:

> When all knots that fetter the heart are cut asunder, then
> a mortal becomes immortal.
> Thus far is the teaching. A hundred and one are the *nāḍīs*
> of the heart,
> one of them leads up to the crown of the head.
> Going upward through that, one becomes immortal.[7]

The Ocean of the Heart

In much of Indian mythology, the ocean is thought to be the source of all life. In the body, the ocean of the heart (*samudra*) is the very source of consciousness and in turn is the origin of the entire phenomenal world.

The metaphor of the ocean of the heart suggests an all-inclusive totality, incorporating everything from the outermost galaxy down to the finest grain of sand. In this sense the ocean of the heart is boundless and immeasurable. The heart is identified with absolute consciousness—inexhaustible, all encompassing, and beyond calculation.

In the ocean of the heart, all arises within the heart like waves on the surface of the ocean. Just as there are myriad peaks and troughs in the waves of the ocean, the heart is the residence of innumerable vicissitudes of feeling. Thus, the all-containing heart as ocean is an all-encompassing singularlity that includes waves of ongoing difference.

PRACTICE

Rolling Waves of Thought on the Ocean of the Heart

This practice is a guide to directly experience the nondual nature of the ocean of the heart. Begin by assuming a comfortable seat on a four- to six-inch support. Note the fluid rhythm of your breath and allow your heart to suspend like a buoy on the tidal movement of breath. Sense the vast, fathomless presence of your heart and allow any thoughts about yesterday, today, or tomorrow to come and go like waves on the surface of your heart-ocean. See that all sensations, perceptions, and thoughts are simply part of the flux of this vast heart-ocean. Do not be consumed by any one particular wave (*ūrmi*) of sensation, perception, or thought. Simply see the fluctuations as part of a great ocean. Observe how any thought formation, after taking shape, dissolves back into the formless ocean. Whether your mind is still or moving, develop conviction that it is all part of one ocean. This is a way to directly perceive the nondual nature of the mind-heart. Stay for fifteen to thirty minutes, and then lie down to rest.

The Great Regulator

In the *Rig Veda*, the oldest collection of stories and verses that explore the ontological origins of being, the heart is mentioned nearly one hundred times. The earliest Sanskrit reference denoting the heart is *hṛd* or *hṛdaya*, which can refer to either mind or heart. Hṛdaya implies the center, essence, or heart of a thing.

It is likely that the English word *heart* derives from the Sanskrit *hṛd*. In Sanskrit, the etymological breakdown of this word *hṛdaya* has interesting correlations to the function of the anatomical heart. The prefix *hṛ* means to remove, and we could think of the blood that flows back to the anatomical heart as being "removed" from the body and carried back to the heart. The Sanskrit syllable *da* means "to give" or offer, and so the heart is the giver, the organ that extends or offers blood to the rest of the body. The final syllable *ya* derives from the root *yam* meaning to regulate, as in the regulatory limbs of Aṣṭāṅga Yoga, the eight-limbed path: *yama* (regulation of conduct in relationship to others), *niyama* (regulation of our interior), and *prāṇāyāma* (the regulation of breath).

Thus, we can think of the heart as the remover, the giver, and the great regulator. In the body it is the great regulator, for it regulates its own local neurological activity via a built-in pacemaker and its sensors govern rhythmic activity in the smallest capillaries of the body's periphery. In order to achieve homeostasis, the heart is continually sensing and adjusting for blood pressure changes from the crown of the head to the heels.

Another way that the heart can be perceived as the regulator is within the hierarchy of the chakras. Located in the middle of the configuration of the classic seven chakras, the heart is the intermediary between the lower three chakras (*mūlādhāra, svādhiṣṭhāna*, and *maṇipūra chakras*) and the upper three (*viśuddha, ājñā*, and *sahasrāra chakras*). Thus, the heart synthesizes and coordinates physiological impulses and spiritual energies related to all other chakras (see fig. 7.5).

The Broken Heart

In the classical teachings on yoga, the heart is thought to be the residence of spirit in the body. In numerous passages in the Bhagavad Gītā, Kṛṣṇa reveals to Arjuna that he is in the heart of all living beings:

> I am the Ātma, Arjuna,
> abiding in the heart of all beings;
> and I am the beginning and the middle
> of beings and the end as well.[8]

This suggests that the ātma, like prāṇa, pervades all space and time and, while everywhere, is most intimately associated with the heart. In the path of bhakti yoga, a yoga that the Gītā inspires, the heart is the source, the epicenter for all things manifest and unmanifest. It is the spiritual axis at the center of the dharma wheel, transporting virtue, divine love, and faith. In the Bhagavad Gītā, Kṛṣṇa stands at the back of Arjuna's war chariot as Arjuna's field guide, guru, divine lord, and friend.

The heart in yoga is the innermost resource for all sentiment, and in the language of devotional yoga, it is the source of compassion and empathetic awareness. We could think of the entire yoga practice as a drive (in keeping with the chariot motif) to generate an all-inclusive heart, the totality of which includes, ironically, pain and violence (Arjuna is confronted by the paradoxical obligation of having to wage war against his teachers, friends, and relatives—veritably a war against himself). While the core teachings of yoga espouse nonviolence, the heart is necessarily the field where both benevolent and malevolent forces get played out. In the Bhagavad Gītā, we see the heart as the "field of the dharma" where trials of duty, karma, right understanding, and faith are learned. The very first line in the Gītā, *dharma kṣetre, kuru kṣetre,* "on the field of the dharma on the field of Kuru [the family lineage]," is akin to the modern-day phrase "theater of war" that refers to the location where great conflict is waged. In the Gītā, this theater of war takes place principally on the stage of the heart. For Arjuna (and the rest of us), the field of the heart is where trials and tribulations of kinship, identity, and selfhood are put to the test.

In the language of the Buddhist teachings, the term "all sentient beings" implies all beings that are conscious and aware, and awareness inevitably involves some degree of suffering. According to the first turning of the wheel of dharma and the initial teachings of Gautama Buddha around the second century C.E., the first of the Four Noble Truths suggests that awakened life inherently includes the experience of suffering. Given this inherent pain, the path of the bodhisattva is to care for all sentient beings, primarily by cultivating greater sympathetic resonance in the heart—feeling for animals, people, the planet, and conditioned experience. The vow of the bodhisattva is a vow of the heart, and, like caring for a garden, the bodhisattva tends to the sorrow and pain that impacts the human heart. This vow requires fortitude and a kind of radical openness to pain. As Trungpa Rinpoche, the founder of Shambhala Buddhist practice in the United States, once said, "Our only weapon is the weapon of gentleness."

At Easter, a similar power and meaning is told of in the heart of the Christian faith. Each year I travel with my family to the Christ in the Desert Monastery, a spectacularly beautiful setting along the Chama River canyon two hours north of Santa Fe, New Mexico, for Easter Mass. The image of the crucified Christ and the precious blood spilled from his feet, hands, and heart suggests an essential, unavoidable pain and suffering intrinsic to all beings. The broken heart epitomizes the pain inherent in our experience of the conditioned world. The heart that suffers is in turn the heart that can truly feel great love and compassion for all beings.

Any dissolution of self in favor of divine union necessitates a breaking open of the heart. The experience of loss and pain, fundamental to all sentient beings in the world, is the gateway to a kind of immersion with the infinite. In the language of classical yoga, this is when the limited, individual self yokes to the vast, unlimited Self, and one who loves unconditionally becomes inseparable from his or her beloved.

The Lotus Heart

The notion that the essential self dwells eternally inside the heart is suggested in a devotional chant to Śiva, dating back to the *Yajurveda*. The verse captures the indivisibility of opposing forces: male and female, active and passive, transcendent and ordinary, and immediate and eternal. It suggests the unity of opposites, particularly the union of Śiva and his consort. The merging of seemingly contradictory entities, which include the two sides of the body, the sun channel (*sūrya nāḍī*) on the right and the lunar channel (*chandra nāḍī*) on the left, is celebrated as "always dwelling in the lotus heart" (*sadā vasantaṃ hṛdayāravinde*). The heart takes the form of a lotus, imbued with devotional sentiment and feelings of profound integration. This integration, a marriage of opposites, leads to a spirit of unconditional acceptance. Like many of the Buddhist and Hindu tantric icons depicting the interpenetration of male and female entities, Śiva and Śakti are described as entwined together. Their joining suggests a kind of endless inter-

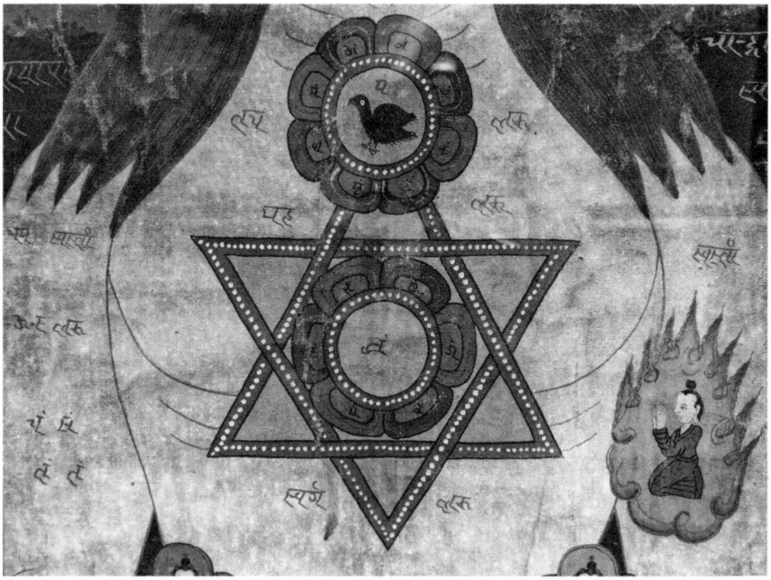

Figure 6.9
Sacred
Hexagram
of the Heart

course, not simply a corporeal conjunction but a metaphysical union, a heart-centered yoga. For it is in the heart that deep affinity and total absorption take place.

This union of opposing energies residing in the heart chakra is symbolically depicted as two equilateral triangles interwoven together. In graphic depictions of the heart chakra, a pair of intertwining triangles overlays the heart center (fig. 6.9). In chapter 3 we examined the integrative power of the Sri Yantra whose multiple interpenetrating triangles are suggestive of all creation (see fig. 3.7). A miniature version of this yantra is the framework for all energies of the heart. This hexagram (*ṣaṭkoṇa*) is the same as the Star of David (or Shield of David) that is recognizable today as the seal of Jewish identity. The six-pointed star radiates in all directions, suggesting the total inclusivity of the heart. In the sacred geometry of the heart chakra, the triangles are superimposed upon a mandala of twelve lotus petals (only six are shown in fig. 6.9). The woven triangles of the heart indicate the heart's capacity to synthesize all bioenergetic currents in the body.

The Heart Chakra and Its Vibration

The physiological and spiritual heart center is referred to as the *hṛt chakra* but is more commonly known as the *anāhata chakra*. The heart is thought to contain a mystical, silent sound that, like the perpetual expansion of the universe, resounds continually. Vibration within the heart is, paradoxically, called the "unstruck sound" (*anāhata śabda*), implying a profound, unruffled stillness. In the depths of meditation, it is possible to experience silence resonating in the heart—a silence purported to lie at the very foundation of being.

In the transformational alchemy of the subtle body, yogis attune to vibration conducted through interior pathways of the body. Sound travels through nāḍīs, and like the vibrating strings of a sitar, pure sound currents reverberate through the nerves and vessels. Thus, frequencies of sound are borne on the prāṇa, moving through the fluids and tissues of the body. When the bones, joints, ligaments, and organs align in āsana and the lungs and heart expand through prāṇāyāma, the "soundless sound" of prāṇa is amplified.

Om is the classic syllabic current used to expand and harmonize the vibratory rhythms of the heart in the subtle body. Throughout the sacred literature of India, the morpheme Om denotes the sound current of the divine (*śabda Brāhma*). In the first chapter of Patañjali's Yoga Sutras, which extolls samādhi, the enunciation of Om, *tasya vācakaḥ praṇavaḥ* (I.27), exalts the divine within by amplifying the inner acoustics of the heart. Thus, it is through sound vibration—sound that eludes the interpretive powers of the intellect—that a divine presence awakens. With this said, the heart is the source of all vibratory rhythm, audible to those who can attune to its sublime presence.

During spells of profound meditation, the atmospheric space of the heart expands and absorbs the mind, the result being an interior state of quiescent joy. In this way, the vibrations of the spiritual heart called *spanda* are inseparable from the flow of consciousness. In the *Vijñāna Bhairava* (Wisdom of Śiva), a collection of tantric teachings from Kashmir compiled around the eighth century C.E., it is said,

He whose mind together with the senses is merged into the
interior space of the heart,
Who has entered mentally into the middle of the heart lotus,
Who has excluded everything else from consciousness,
Acquires the highest fortune.[9]

PRACTICE

The Flame of the Heart Meditation

The aim of this heart meditation is to cultivate undistracted awareness and interior light by imagining a steady flame in the cave of your heart.

Begin by sitting comfortably on a three- to six-inch support and releasing the weight of your leg bones and pelvis into the cushion. Lift the sides of your trunk and raise and open the region around the *eyes of your heart.* Close your eyes and visualize a flame in the middle of the cave of your heart. As you settle into a very light rhythm with your breath, imagine this heart flame burning steadily. Should winds of distraction penetrate your heart-mind, then the flame will waver, flicker, and burn uncontrollably. When distracted the flame will not burn brightly and its oscillations will cause the flame tip to smoke, clouding your concentration. Make your breath even, soft, and steady. This will help the flame of your heart burn steadfast and still. Visualize an unruffled flame with a constant glow, like a flame in a windless place. Imagine the radiance and glow of this steady light filling your entire chest. Sense the spirit of great joy that accompanies this unperturbed, undying flame within. Remain for five to forty-five minutes.

The Cave of the Heart

One of the common allusions to the heart in yoga metaphysics is that of the heart as a cave. Hidden, secret, and inscrutable, the heart is like an ancient grotto wherein the lantern of awareness is kept lit.

As a way of describing entry into the cave of the heart, from surface to depth, my Dzogchen teacher in Tibetan Buddhist practice,

Tsoknyi Rinpoche, outlines three aspects of the heart—the outer, inner, and secret (innermost) heart. The outer heart can be thought of as the threshold to the cave. It is affected by circumstances and interactions with people—in a sense, it is shaped by the day-to-day effects of karma. Any formulation of a social self is determined by exchanges and contacts that occur at the level of the outer heart. This layer is a source of both joy and pain, as thoughts, emotions, hopes, and fears are conditioned by outside phenomena. The outer heart is subject to the variable winds of circumstance, and as a result, confusion, anger, attachment, pride, and jealousy (the five poisons) can metastasize inside.

The inner heart, the second layer, is located in the interior heart cave. It is a repository for our inner feelings, moods, and impressions. This middle heart holds the personal sense of *I,* born from myriad imprints that determine how we feel about ourselves. This includes everything that is ingrained in the psyche due to conditioning, initially and formatively, by the domestic scene into which we are born. It includes self-image; thoughts, judgments, habitual affect, and personal identity. This layer has lasting, hidden, often ambiguous effects on the subtle body.

The deepest level, the secret heart, has an affinity with the immeasurable—that which cannot be put into language and can never be known. This secret heart is intimately woven within the subtle body. Due to its depth, it can never be named or recognized. The only way to commune with this deep-seated, enduring heart is by moving into the deep recesses of the cave, veritably a journey into the heart of darkness. This move involves a radical suspension of self, a direct experience of utter selflessness. Since thought, cognition, and intellect are barred from gaining access to the secret heart (like Plato's shadows, they merely project traces of their own images), the ultimate way to arrive at this layer is through unmitigated surrender, a kind of out-and-out, total letting go. By ceding to not knowing, by capitulating to the darkest recesses of the heart cave, we "see the greatness of the self, [our] sorrow at an end."[10] In Buddhist teaching, this unforgettable dropping away of self-identity is described as *śūnyatā* (emptiness). My Zen teacher Roshi Joan Sutherland identifies this journey into the wisdom of the subtle body and the depth of the heart as the process of "endarkenment."

PRACTICE

Meditation in the Cave of the Heart

This meditation guides one to the very depths of the interior heart, to the secret heart, a place beyond comprehension that transcends linguistic reference. Assume a comfortable seated position and begin your session with soft, slow strokes of your breath. Settle into the weight of your bones and be sure to relax your jaw, tongue, and throat. Gently shepherd your awareness into the cave of your heart. Become aware of the outside surface of your anatomical heart, the side that faces outward toward the world. In so doing, recall any events within the last several hours, days, or weeks that have had an impact on your emotional being. Make note of the events or the people that form the constellation of your felt experience in this outer heart.

Next, bring awareness to your inner heart and notice how outside circumstances affect your breathing, heart rate, brain waves, and electrical signals. This involves the process of interoception, observing feelings of pain, body temperature, pulsation, tingling, and so forth. These sensations may reflect emotive states of humiliation, judgment, shame, irritation, intolerance, and so on. Notice how there may be traces of toxic feeling left in your subtle body from events or personal relationships that have arisen in your life. Be patient and tolerant while practicing nonjudgmental awareness.

Finally, bring awareness to the posterior surface of your heart, the side that faces inward toward your spine. This is the secret heart that is outside karma, outside of circumstances, causes, and conditions. Conjure feelings of space and lightness in this innermost recess of your heart. Avoid attempting to identify or make cognitive sense of your experience. With undistracted awareness, allow yourself to be absorbed into your secret heart and into silence, space, and a sense of timelessness. This realm is uncontaminated by bias, interpretation, or judgment. Rest your awareness in the unspeakable, unintelligible, and truly vast realm of your innermost heart. Remain for ten to thirty minutes.

7

BLUE THROAT

The Confluence of Many Rivers

Śiva, Supreme above all, yours is the beginning, yours is the first fruit of everything. Only you can drink Kālakuta, *the poison of the world . . . Only he who assimilates the poison of the world will have the strength of compassion.*

—Roberto Calasso, *Ka: Stories of the Mind and Gods of India*[1]

To prepare the mind for subtle states of meditative awareness and samādhi, classical yoga places great importance on bringing space and relaxation to the throat and neck. Structurally this is not easy because in the uppermost chest, the torso makes an abrupt transition as it funnels into the neck. In the way that ships pass from the Atlantic to the Pacific through the straits of the Panama Canal, large amounts of blood and numerous nerves channel through the neck, connecting the brain and trunk. For this reason, the neck is vulnerable to congestion, and the delicate vertebrae, small muscles, and highly mobile joints within the neck are vulnerable to torque, twist, and displacement. Given the fragility and highly sensitive nature of its vessels, glands, and nerves, the neck and throat together are a common repository for strain. Veritably, this area is a potential perfect storm, for not only is it prone to musculoskeletal strain but due to its proximity to the brain it is vulnerable to the high winds of psychological tension. It is common for emotional turbulence including worry, anxiety, and fear to constrict the throat. Traditional yoga practices make us aware that the throat chakra is a critical conjunction of energetic forces, and only by unbottling the neck can prāṇa in the subtle body flow unconstrained.

The neck is in the precarious role of bridging the heart and the head. The throughway of the neck is responsible for helping establish congruity, both physiologically and emotionally, between the sentiment center of the heart and the cognitive center of the brain. The alignment of heart and head, celebrated in contemplative Buddhist practices as the balance of wisdom and compassion, requires profound and ongoing integration. Integrating thought with feeling is not an easy task. Additionally the throat, intermediary between heart and head, is the locus for vocalization and self-expression.

It is a common assumption that structurally, the throat is limited to the area just below the jaw and is only several inches in length. Yet we can imagine the throat chakra to be far more extensive, if we consider its range from the roof of the mouth to the diaphragm. The pharynx includes the windpipe (the trachea) and the tube that transports food from mouth to stomach (the esophagus). The upper margin of the throat cavity includes the palate, nasal septum, and opening to the auditory tubes. The lower border is the respiratory diaphragm. This range of the throat suggests its extensive influence on the body.

The neck is unique and complex, a narrow region that houses a series of overlapping cylinders: the trachea (respiratory tract), the esophagus (digestive tract), and the spinal cord (neurological tract). The upper palate is the confluence of these systems and it plays a critical role in the chakra system. It is not only the roof of the throat chakra but the gateway into the sublime interior channel, the *suṣumnā*.

In this chapter we explore the vital and delicate throat center in a variety of ways. We will review the numerous cleansing and purifying practices within haṭha yoga involving the tongue, nasal passages, tonsils, and vocal cords. We explore the many ways that the throat is vulnerable to tension and how winds of distress can cause constriction. In the practice of yoga postures and in the movement of jālandhara bandha, we will aim to relax the throat, tongue, jaw, and neck muscles. Finally, we will examine how in the esoteric language of yoga, mythic drops of immortality (*amṛta*) are thought to drip down from the skull. It is paramount that the yogi, by creating an internal seal in the well of the throat, deftly catches the precious droplets before they descend into the gastric fires of his mortal body.

Throat Purification

In many ways, the aim of haṭha yoga is to provide a cleansing and purgative effect on the entire body-mind, particularly within the throat region, given that it is a high-risk area for infection. This emphasis on purity is prioritized in the overall path of Aṣṭāṅga Yoga, as cleanliness (*śauca*) appears as the first of the *niyamas* (internal disciplines). One of the hallmarks of yoga and Āyurveda is health of the physical body so that further transformation can occur in the more delicate subtle body.

Along the banks of the neck and scattered throughout the throat region is a trellis of lymph nodes. Part of the fluid system, the cervical nodes provide a crucial line of defense against invasive bacteria that might enter the body through the nostrils, ears, and oral cavity. Chains of lymph vessels and nodes line the tongue, jaw, pharynx, esophagus, and trachea. Like sentinels guarding the primary entry ports to a city, lymph vessels monitor the flow of any unwanted particulates. Specialized lymph structures at the back of the oral cavity—the uvula, tonsils, and adenoids—provide the first line of defense. In the chakra system, the name for the throat chakra is directly relevant to the immune system. The *viśuddha chakra* comes from the Sanskrit verbal root *śud,* meaning to cleanse or purify, so *viśuddha* translates as "in-depth purification." If the throat is the body's primary barrier relating to immunity, how does yogic practice aid this process of purification?

One of the practices that most defines yoga is nasal breathing.

Nasal breathing sets yoga apart from other physical training such as athletics, gymnastics, and ballet where competitors never consider breathing through their nose. Given that the nasal apertures are narrower than the mouth, nostril breathing requires concentration on the breath, as outside air is siphoned as it flows into the labyrinthine nasal passages. As the breath circulates through the nasal cavities, nostril hairs warm and filter the air, reducing the chance of bacterial or viral encroachment. *Ujjāyī* breath, where the breath is siphoned in the back of the throat, is the most accessible of all prāṇāyāmas and the first type of prāṇāyāma to learn. Other prāṇāyāmas serve to "dry clean" the throat. *Kapālabhāti* (skull-shining breath), which is done by pumping the abdomen in and out like a bellows, is thought to eradicate mucous disorders of the throat. *Nāḍī śodhana* (alternate-nostril breath) serves to sanitize and "polish" the prāṇa as it flows in through the nostrils. Nāḍī śodhana prāṇāyāma also acts as a kind of nasal wash. This is suggested by the word *śodhana,* which has the same verbal root as the word *viśuddha, śud* meaning to wash or cleanse.

Another common technique used to cleanse the throat chakra and the nasopharynx is *neti,* a process whereby water is funneled (sometimes with herbs) through the nose and out the mouth in order to evacuate the nasal sinuses and keep them clear. Also, *nasya,* part of the protocol for *pañchakarma* in Āyurveda, is prescribed for bodily purification. It involves nasal administration of medicated oil. In times before dentists and electric toothbrushes, these various techniques for rinsing the back of the oral cavity helped prevent not only sinus congestion but also tonsillitis and respiratory infection. It is said in the *Haṭha Yoga Pradīpikā*:

> Neti (nasal rinse) cleanses the cranium
> And bestows clairvoyance.
> It also destroys all diseases
> Which manifest above the throat.[2]

More extreme forms of oral-nasal cleansing involve threading a cloth string between the nostrils and mouth in order to floss the nasal passages, or swallowing a wet cloth as far as the stomach (both called *dhauti,* which means internal cleansing). You might wonder if these last two techniques will lead to clairvoyance or a headache. In any event, internal cleansing practices in yoga recommend regularly rinsing and flushing the membranes of the nostrils and throat.

Of all the myriad poses in yoga, sarvangāsana (shoulderstand) and halāsana (plow pose) are the essential poses to flush the lymph nodes and vessels of the throat. Due to its nourishing effects, the shoulderstand is called "the mother of all poses." It is thought to have curative and replenishing effects on the throat chakra—on the nasopharynx, thyroid and parathyroid glands, lymph nodes, and tongue. However, since shoulderstand and plow require balancing on the shoulders, rigidity and muscular tension in the shoulders and upper trunk make them difficult to perform.

Sarvangāsana supports drainage of blood and lymph out of the legs, gut, and chest. Lymph collectors throughout the body transport lymph to terminal pathways deep in the venous system at the base of the neck. Since lymph flows in little waves via peristaltic contractions, local pressure serves to squeeze or "milk" the lymphatic ducts. In shoulderstand, the combination of full diaphragmatic breathing (which also helps drive the lymph) and weight on the shoulder girdle helps irrigate lymph through superficial epidermal layers and deep visceral layers of the body.

When performing shoulderstand, it is essential that there is only light pressure on the throat and neck (it is not a neck stand!), since optimal lymph drainage happens as a result of a gentle compressive force. Akin to the squeegee-like mechanism of a sponge mop, when lymphatic vessels are compressed they respond with greater contractile, secretory, and absorptive capacities. In shoulderstand, undue weight on the neck (as is likely for students who do not correctly support their shoulders) can inhibit the pulsatory flow of lymph and also aggravate the cervical vertebrae, intervertebral disks, and related spinal nerves.

Prāṇa Pollution

Yoga techniques that serve to flush the delicate membranes of the nostrils and throat are invaluable today in light of atmospheric pollution. An abundance of airborne particulates swirl through the skies including dust, dirt, aerosols, smoke, pollen, and pollutants. Due to exposure to contaminants, respiratory conditions such as allergies, asthma, and chronic obstructive pulmonary disease (COPD) are on the rise. In cities all over the world, the air is plagued with high levels of fine particulates that are considered unsafe to breathe. Yoga poses and cleansing techniques that bathe the respiratory tract and boost the immune system help to counter the effects of respiratory inflammation.

PRACTICE

Shoulderstand, the Mother of All Poses

It is important to perform shoulderstands on a supportive platform to avoid excessive pressure on the neck. Choose a support that is soft but firm; a stack of blankets four- to six-inches high is preferable, or you can use a bolster that is neither too rigid nor squishy.

Lie on your back and place your shoulders at the edge of the platform in such a way that your head is below the level of your shoulders on the floor. Pin your arms to the platform along the sides of your hips and swing your legs up. Either move into halāsana (plow pose) or swing straight up into sarvāngāsana (shoulderstand). If you can perform plow pose, revolve the outer edge of your shoulders underneath you as if you are tucking a fitted sheet under the corner of a mattress. This will insure that your weight is resting on your shoulder blades and not your neck. Once you have revolved your shoulders underneath you, step up into shoulderstand one leg at a time.

In shoulderstand, comfort is the key, so avoid placing undue pressure on your neck or head. You should not feel excessive pressure in your ears or eyes. Observe that the majority of your weight falls on the uppermost edge of your shoulder blades (called the spine of the scapulae). To accomplish this, press your hands firmly into your back ribs and actively extend your legs upward from your pelvis. If you find that the weight falls on your neck, then your elbows are too far apart. You may want to loop a strap just above your elbows to hold your upper arms parallel to each other.

There are five ways to orient your legs to help defray tension from your neck. These variations also serve to release pressure in the pelvic floor. Stay for approximately one minute in each variation: (1) legs extended, inner feet together, (2) feet hip-distance apart, (3) feet as wide apart as your mat, (4) feet apart as in *upaviṣṭa koṇāsana* (wide-angle pose), and (5) feet in baddha koṇāsana (bound angle pose). All the while be sure to keep your sacral region lifted and your throat and tongue soft. Stay three to seven minutes in total. From shoulderstand release your legs back to plow pose and then slowly lower your legs without lifting your head. Lie for a minute in śavāsana with your knees bent.

Jālandhara Bandha

In addition to postures and cleansing techniques for the throat, *jālandhara bandha*, the "throat seal," regulates the blood, lymph, and nerve impulses that pass through the neck. Anatomically, jālandhara bandha seals off the membranous sheathing of the vocal cords—two slender V-shaped flaps. The larynx houses the vocal cords, delicate triangular folds that are the source of oral expression. Located just below the glottis and just above the butterfly-shaped thyroid, the voice box is approximately two centimeters wide, lined with mucus, and the size and consistency of a ripe apricot. If you place your fingers on your Adam's apple, called the thyroid cartilage, the vocal cords are located just behind this barrier. Here in the tenuous cavity of the larynx, prāṇa and sound unite (fig. 7.1).

Figure 7.1
The Palate and Throat Chakra

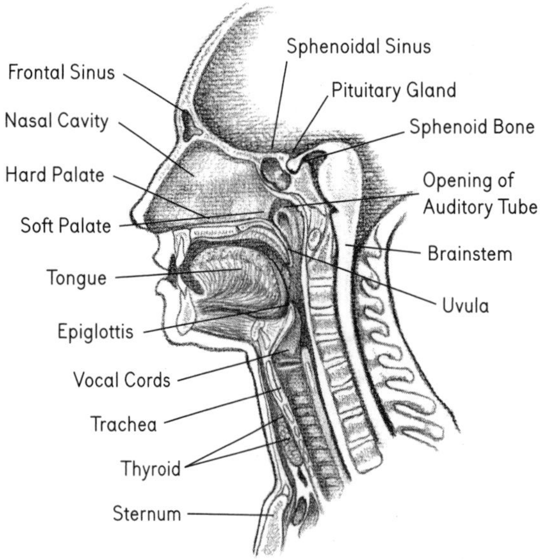

The vocal cords form an operable mini-diaphragm, our fourth horizontal sheathing in the body (see fig. 8.4). When they are apart and relaxed, they allow air to pass. When they are pulled taut and drawn together, they close. When air is expelled through the cords it vibrates and produces sound, in the way that air escaping from the nozzle of a held balloon creates a high-pitch trill. In order to regulate the flow of air into the lungs, yogis partially seal off this vocal diaphragm by retracting the chin and moving it downward. This seal is responsible for generating the sound of ujjāyī breath.

Just as mūla bandha moniters the opening and closing of the perineum and uḍḍīyāna bandha monitors the opening and closing of the respiratory diaphragm, jālandhara bandha regulates the opening and closing of the vocal cord diaphragm. Done together, these three bandhas create *mahā bandha* (the great seal), which is thought to amplify the flow of prāṇa through the subtle body.

Jālandhara bandha is done by folding the chin down against the elevated sternum. This movement is difficult to perform given the structural and psychological tension so pervasive in the neck region. Fishing birds such as cormorants, pelicans, geese, and cranes demonstrate this fold via remarkably elastic neck pouches used for nabbing prey and draining water. Fishing birds are considered to be sacred in Japanese, Chinese, and Indian mythology, celebrated for their capacity to both swim in water (signifying immersion in the world of temporality and flux) and fly in the sky (signifying travel in the heavenly or formless realm). There are yoga poses named for long-necked, long-legged water fowl—*krauñcāsana* (heron pose) and bakāsana (crane pose)—and in tai chi and qigong entire movements are attributed to the graceful, concentrated, and poised movements of the crane.

The word *jālandhara* relates to a fishing bird, for *jāla* means net or sieve, suggesting the retractable throat pouch of a great blue heron or pelican. *Jālandhara bandha* is often mistranslated as "throat lock," but it more accurately suggests a colander-like function where fluids are filtered as they pass between the chest cavity and cranium. Drawing the chest and chin toward each other stimulates the lymph vessels, mucous membranes, and blood vessels, and helps siphon out debris or toxins. By tucking the mandible down, the fleshy tissues of the throat plexus—thyroid, parathyroid gland, hyoid muscles, and lymph ducts—are vicariously squeezed and flushed.

The movement of jālandhara bandha gently squeezes or "milks" the butterfly-shaped thyroid gland located in the throat (see figs. 6.7 and 7.1). Along with the intracranial glands (pituitary and pineal), the thyroid is one of the master glands of the body, and the yogis knew intuitively that its hormonal secretions have powerful effects on the subtle body (*śukra dhātu*). The regulatory rhythms of the thyroid contribute to overall vitality, as thyroxin secreted out of the thyroid monitors tissue metabolism. Thyroid function has significant control over our body clock and is partly responsible for what makes us tick. The thyroid does not act in isolation, for it is constantly "texting" the adrenals and pituitary in order to monitor overall energy levels in the body. The internal effects of shoulderstand, plow, and jālandhara bandha stimulate the thyroid's glandular secretions and regulate its complex rhythms.

Done in combination with prāṇāyāma and *pratyāhāra* (interiorizing the senses), jālandhara bandha helps lower blood pressure and increase parasympathetic activity. In jālandhara bandha, the forward nodding of the head involves a shift in blood pressure within the cerebral nerve centers in the brain. If you have ever felt faint or light-headed, you may recall having lowered your head. This reflex is a protective response triggered by the autonomic nervous system responsible for modulating blood pressure, heart rate, and vascular tone. During jālandhara bandha, the autonomic centers in the brain stem receive signals from baroreceptors in the carotid arteries and the aorta to monitor blood pressure. With the head folded down over the crease of the neck, the brain moves partially into energy-conserving mode. Lowering the head increases parasympathetic activity in the vagus nerve that transits through the neck, prompting feelings of calm and serenity. Combined with full diaphragmatic breathing, jālandhara bandha serves to decrease heart rate, blood pressure, and rate of respiration.

Initially it is best to learn jālandhara bandha by regularly practicing shoulderstands and plow pose, for these positions help create the seal between the chest and chin. In shoulderstand the vocal diaphragm, thyroid, surrounding cartilage, and musculature are pressurized, making the throat pouch more elastic. Many students develop an antipathy for these poses due to feelings of suffocation and confinement. Initially I recommend that students learn shoulderstands with their feet against a wall and shins parallel to the floor to ensure that there is not excessive pressure on their neck.

PRACTICE

Preparation for Jālandhara Bandha

This exercise prepares your neck and throat for jālandhara bandha. Lie on your back and set a block on its flat side underneath the back of your head. With your head propped, the back of your neck will lengthen as your chin draws down toward your sternum. Be sure that your throat remains soft and without strain. Bring your arms down by your sides, clasp the side of the mat with your hands and pull. This will help pin your shoulders down and away from the back of your skull. At the same time, roll your outer shoulders into the floor to broaden your sternum and collarbones. Be sure that your throat remains soft. Hold this position for three minutes.

Come out of the pose and while still on your back, loop one end of an eight-foot long strap over the base of your skull (it should set like a mini-harness over your occiput). Bend your knees into your chest and loop the other end of the strap over your feet. Slowly extend your legs toward the ceiling to place tension on the strap. The strap sling will pull your head into flexion, thereby tractioning the muscles at the base of your skull (upper trapezius, longissimus dorsi, semispinalis, and suboccipital muscles). Remain for several minutes.

Come out of the pose and move into halāsana (plow pose) followed by sarvangāsana (shoulderstand), following the instructions for the "Mother of All Poses" exercise earlier in this chapter. As you invert your torso, be sure to keep your throat soft and notice the way your sternum and chin are brought close together.

Finally, come to a seated position with the sides of your trunk elevated and the top two corners of your chest (the "eyes of the heart") lifted and open. Gently bring your chin down while sliding the back of your skull upward. At the same time, raise your breastbone so that your sternum spreads both vertically and horizontally. Then, wedge a washcloth or very small towel between your sternum and chin. This will enable you to yoke your chest and chin together in the seal of jālandhara bandha without having to force or cram your head downward. The downward movement of your head should induce feelings of quiet and serenity. Turn your awareness to your inhalation, filling your lungs slowly. At this point, you can practice the Viloma I prāṇāyāma described in chapter 6.

The Atlas's Heavy Load

The transition from the neck to the skull is a critical juncture in terms of spinal dynamics and the overall balance of the viśuddha chakra. It is valuable to regard the throat chakra as involving not only the structures anterior to the cervical spine but also the posterior neck together with the cranial base. The uppermost vertebrae are not secured together like the lumbar vertebrae in the lower back. While the lumbar vertebrae are interlocked by sturdy facet joints that provide a stout and stable base, the cervical vertebrae are free to move. As a result, the cervical vertebrae can articulate with greater range of motion than the lumbar vertebrae. The neck can side bend and rotate enabling the skull on top of the first cervical vertebrae to freely nod "yes," shake "no," or swivel in multiple directions.

Generally, the greater the potential range of movement in the body, the greater the likelihood of dysfunction. This is certainly the case for the juncture of the first cervical vertebra and skull (called the atlanto-occipital joint, or AO joint). We saw earlier how the base of the spinal column at the lumbar-sacral junction is vulnerable to routine strain and compression; in a reciprocal way, the apex of the vertebral column at the cranial-spinal junction is prone to displacement.

The first cervical vertebra (C1) is called the atlas, so named for the Greek god who hoisted the world on his upper back and shoulders. The atlas bone's Herculean task of propping up the cranial globe frequently results in buckling and shearing that cause the AO joint to displace. All too often the cranium does not perch symmetrically atop the spine, and most people literally do not have their head on straight. Usually the problem involves unilateral musculoskeletal adhesions—

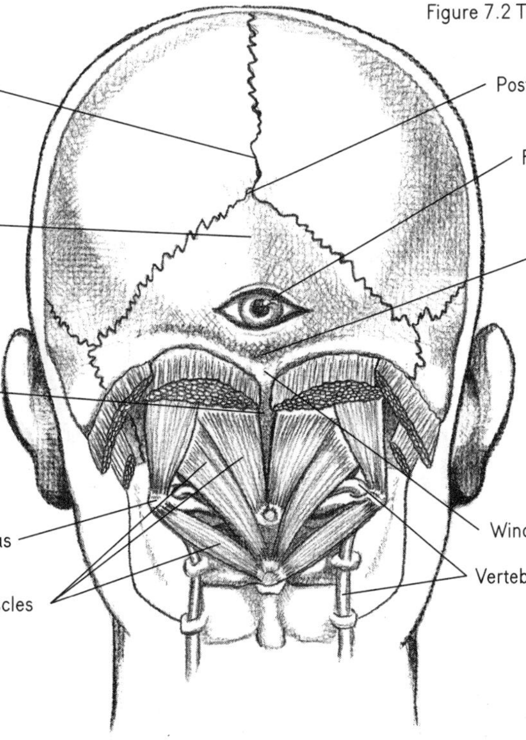

Figure 7.2 The Cervical-Cranial Juncture

that is, the neck pitches to one side due to tension in the soft tissues along the side of the neck. The small suboccipital muscles are inevitably involved. Notice how these muscles orient vertically, diagonally, and (nearly) horizontally, enabling the cranium to swivel on the first cervical vertebrae in numerous ways (fig. 7.2).

Due to right-handedness and right-shoulder dominance, it is common for the right side of the neck to be taut, pulling the right ear down toward the right shoulder. This may be coupled with strain in the right shoulder, adhesions in the right arm or hand, and irritation in the right eye. In the language of yoga, this right-side compression is identified as inflammation of the dominant "solar" side of the body (*piṅgalā nāḍī*). When the right side of skull tips and collapses to the right, the atlas slides left.

The occipital bone at the back of the skull is held aloft via two small

Figure 7.3 Occipital Condyles, Cranial "Heels"

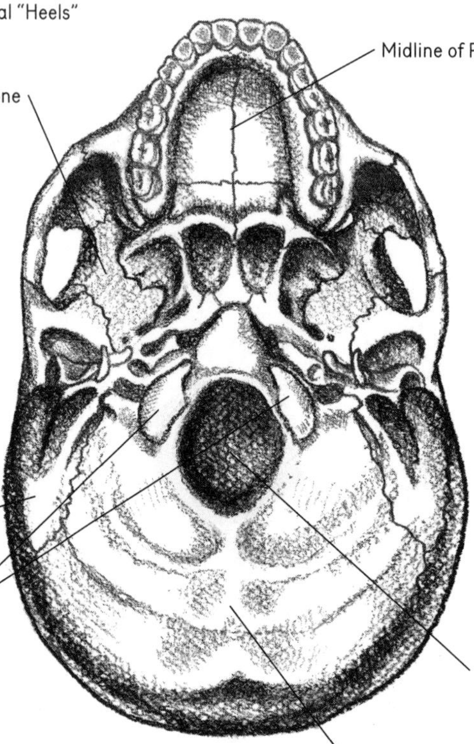

feet planted on the atlas. They are called occipital condyles, and I think of them as the sitting bones of the cranium (fig. 7.3). They are our third set of heels, the first being the heels of the feet, and the second being the heels of the buttock bones (see fig. 2.4). In order to achieve stability and levity in virtually all of the poses, these three sets of heels must align and be balanced. In order for a pose to be stable and harmonious, what Patañjali defined in the Yoga Sutras as *sthira sukham āsanam,* alignment within these three sets of heels is necessary. Balancing the skull on its cranial heels enables optimal circulation of blood and nerve impulses into the skull. This includes the vertebral arteries that thread through the narrow processes of the cervical vertebrae. Along with the carotid arteries, the vertebral arteries are the only other arteries to supply blood to the brain (see fig. 7.2). Aligning the cranial base requires ongoing care and practice because it is common for dysfunction to occur in the simplest of activities—sleeping, talking on the phone, carrying a backpack, and so on.

PRACTICE

Balancing the Pelvic and Cranial Heels

This exercise aligns the contact points of your sitting bones (the pelvic heels) with the base of your skull, the occipital condyles (the cranial heels). This practice may give you a sense as to whether one side of your neck is more restricted than the other.

Assume a comfortable sitting position and make sure your sitting bones are balanced. Once you settle into your cushion, slowly rock from side to side on your sitting bones. Make the swaying movement as small and discreet as possible. Notice which sitting bone makes better contact with your cushion and which side of your lower back may be tighter than the other. Then align to the midline equidistant between your sitting bones. Position your skull directly over your pelvis so that your head is not pulling to the right or left, nor falling forward or backward. Gently raise the back of your skull as if you are lifting an antenna to get good reception. The updraft of your occipital base should encourage your entire skull to float. At the same time, dissolve any tension in your jaw, tongue, and face. With a small, soft, barely discernible motion, bob your head from side to side so that you rock on the heels of your occipital condyles. Observe any slight pull or restriction on either side of your neck. Which side of your upper neck is tighter? Then, rest in the midpoint equidistant between your two occipital condyles. In this meditation, the smaller the movement, the more information you will receive about subtle structural biases in your neck and pelvis.

Now rock your weight onto one sitting bone and at the same time lift *the same side* occiput upward toward the ceiling. Notice the polarity between the "heel" of the right sitting bone and the "heel" of your right occipital condyle (they move away from each other); repeat on the other side. After this exploration, pause in the middle and orient to the middle channel of your spine from sacrum to occiput. Hold for three to five minutes before resting in śavāsana for several minutes.

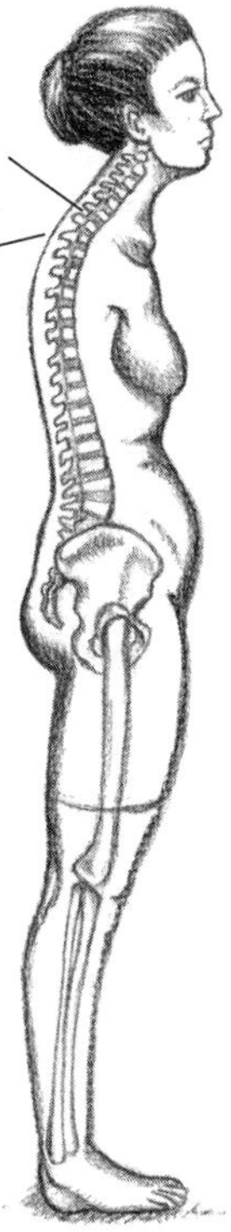

Figure 7.4 Kyphosis of the Upper Back

Hazards of No-Neck-Āsana

The collective structures in the cranium and neck are extremely delicate and are prone to dysfunction. This is partly due to the fact that the head and neck are situated farthest from the ground and like a child's stack of building blocks, the upper mass is vulnerable to sway and topple.

It is most common for the head to lurch forward, creating tension at the base of the neck. This causes the upper thoracic vertebrae to pull backward into an unsightly bulge (fig. 7.4), distorting the cervical-thoracic junction. This is called a dowager's hump, and kyphotic curvature in the lower cervical region is particularly common among the elderly. Today, in the culture of the keyboard when people spend as much as ten hours a day typing at a computer, the shoulders and head drift forward of the midline, contributing to the backward displacement of the upper trunk. As a result, people who log long hours at a desk are more prone to kyphotic curvature earlier in life.

As people age, they inevitably shrink in stature, and nowhere in the body are the results more devastating than in the neck. My Rolfing instructor Jan Sultan used to say in his acerbic, forthright way, "You gotta have a neck," suggesting the importance of length and range of motion of the cervical spine. One of his primary aims as a manual therapist is to promote greater length and space in and around the cranial base. Many people suffer from "no-neck-āsana," meaning that the shoulders shrug upward as the back of the skull slides downward, compacting the neck. In every yoga posture it is critical to create length in the neck while balancing the shoulder girdle efficiently atop the torso.

We saw earlier the difficulty in maintaining integrity at the spinal transitions where posterior curves change direction and become anterior curves. This holds true for the transition between the posterior curve of the occiput and the anterior curve of the neck and the transition between the lower cervical spine and upper thoracic spine (the C7-T1, junction). In order to prevent posterior rounding at C7-T1, one of my yoga teachers described a C7 "bandha," that is, to hold the cervical-thoracic junction firmly in place so the neck retains its length and elegance.

When the upper back displaces backward, the skull loses critical support along with its vertical positioning atop the spine. This affects the body's overall health and longevity. The vital structures that pass through the narrow corridor of the neck are also affected: cervical nerve roots may become impinged and intervertebral disks compressed. Trigger points (TPs) in the musculature of the shoulder and neck can exacerbate this, especially TPs in the upper trapezius muscles. The forward pitch of the head can cause pressure around the brain stem, potentially inhibiting neurological flow through the sixteen cranial nerves that emerge at the cranial base.

Numerous poses help to anchor the scapulae onto the back and relieve the burden of an overwhelmed cervical-thoracic junction. One of the best poses to counter a C curve in the upper back is supported matsyāsana (fish pose) done with a blanket roll or a block wedged under the upper back (see chapter 6 for Supported Fish Pose). By regularly pinning the shoulder blades onto the back by applying mechanical pressure—poses I refer to as "scap traps"—the frontal chest is able to expand while the mass of knotted muscular tension in the upper back dissolves.

PRACTICE

Simple Scap Traps

These exercises are accessible antidotes for people with anterior drag of the shoulders, bound pectoral muscles, and curvature in the upper spine (see figs. 6.5 and 7.4).

1. Stand in tāḍāsana. Clasp the loop of a strap in your hands behind you and actively reach your arms backward away from your trunk. If you have stiff shoulders and cannot straighten your arms, widen the loop. When you grip the strap, turn the palm of each hand outward so that your arms are in external rotation. Continue to hold the strap firmly, raise your side waist, and actively lift your sternum. Stay for one minute and do not let your arms go to sleep.

2. For those who can get down onto the floor, proceed to do supported fish pose from the last chapter. Otherwise, sit on a folding chair facing forward and drape a blanket over the backrest of the chair. Lean back and hook your scapulae against the chair

back. Be sure to pin some part of your shoulder blades, preferably the lower border of your scapula, onto the backrest of the chair. Then clasp your hands to the sides of the chair and pull. Actively broaden your upper ribs and collarbones, while elevating the front of your spine toward the ceiling. Continue to arch your sternum up and back without lifting your pelvis off the seat. The backrest of the chair should act as a fulcrum to help pin your scapulae onto your back. Hold for one minute or more.

Then sit up straight in the chair, facing forward, and interlock your fingers behind you (or use the strap as you did a moment ago). Set your forearms onto the back of the chair. Press down with your forearms as you draw your shoulder blades down and away from the back of your skull. Actively raise your sternum and breathe into your frontal ribs. In this movement your shoulder blades should retract downward and press forward into your body, thus countering excessive posterior thoracic curvature. Hold the pose for a minute or more.

Corresponding Chakras: The Throat and Belly

We explored earlier how chakras at opposing ends of the spine correspond. We saw how the nadir in the mūlādhāra chakra (the root chakra) correlates with the sahasrāra at the top of the head, and how the svādhiṣṭhāna chakra (the second chakra at the sacrum) reciprocates with the forehead and occipital chakra, the ājñā chakra. In this section, we will look further into how the maṇipūra chakra (the third chakra at the digestive center) pairs with the viśuddha chakra (the throat chakra), sharing both physiological and emotional connections (fig. 7.5).

Anatomically the gut and throat are connected via the length of the alimentary canal. Each center is vulnerable to emotional strain, as trapped pain in the body gnaws away at the delicate structures of both belly and throat. Hormonally the adrenal glands in the third chakra and the thyroid gland in the fifth chakra are intricately linked. The thyroid governs the body's overall metabolic function: it is essentially what makes us hum, as it regulates the output of energy. The adrenal glands meanwhile release stress hormones that tell the body how quickly and with what level of energy to respond. Thus, the adrenal-thyroid feed-

Figure 7.5 Chakra Polarities

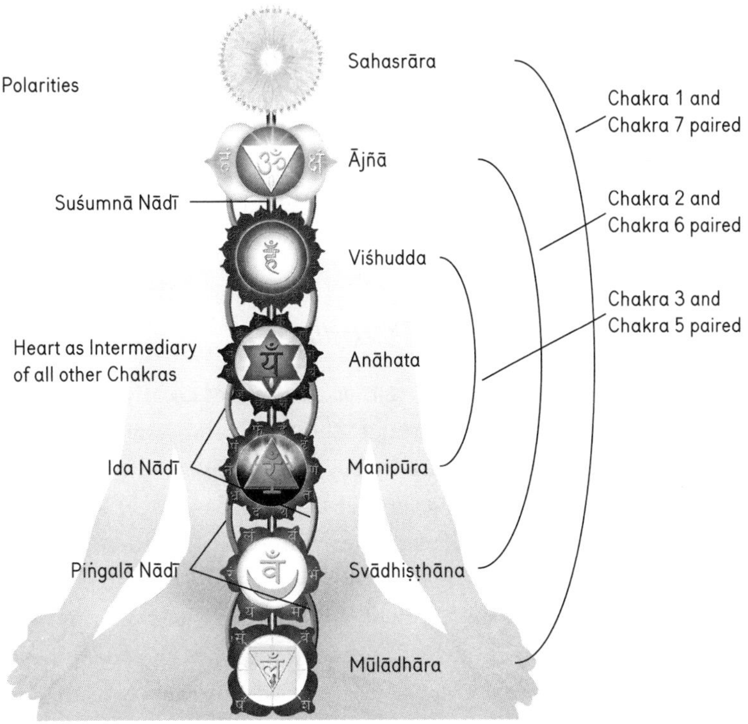

back loop is critical as it dictates the response time and degree of exertion necessary at any given time. Levels of cortisol, a stress hormone, are regulated by the thyroid-adrenal regulatory mechanism.

Fatigue and Thyroid Imbalance

In the language of yoga, the adrenal-thyroid circuit governs the deep life-force (śakti) necessary for leaning forward into the world and taking action. When people are depleted by fatigue, the adrenal-thyroid balance (including glandular secretions from the pituitary and hypothalamus within the brain) are thrown off resulting in hypothyroidism. Low energy, weight gain, depression, constipation, muscle and joint pain, and susceptibility to infection are some of the symptoms related to a hypothyroid condition. Adrenal exhaustion and hypothyroidism weaken the body's overall vitality, its prāṇa śakti.

Together the belly and throat centers oversee the body's sense of command and authority. We know that the third chakra is the seat of the body's biological will, given the survival impulse activated within the adrenal cortex. Similarly, the throat is a resource for power, as speech is the primary command center to express intent, need, and vision. Speech is a critical means to self-expression and to actualizing personal power.

Right Speech, Right Listening

Speech can be either a source of creative self-empowerment, a means to express feelings, thoughts, and visions, or a weapon that divides, degrades, and destroys. At the outset of the eight-limbed path of Patañjali, *satya* (mindful usage of language) appears as a cornerstone of the discipline. In the greater yoga tradition, yoga is simply described as the refinement of body, speech, and mind. Mindful speech (in the Eightfold Path of Buddhism called Right Speech) is not something we typically regard as an essential part of the yoga undertaking, given yoga's current emphasis on physical prowess, breath, and healing emotional wounds. However, considerate speech is a hallmark for monitoring thought, action, and behavior and for gaining access to the subtle body.

Considerate listening requires attention to our inner speech—to thoughts, moods, attitudes, hopes, and fears. In the meditative arts, this is accomplished by spending days, months, and years with sitting bones parked on the meditation cushion. By recognizing inner speech, we begin to interrupt the "habit narrative."

A practice of interior listening aids in the process of sorting through the multitude of voices that get recorded and stored in the psyche over the course of a lifetime. Inculcated voices—the voices of parents, siblings, coaches, and teachers—can be either condemning and degrading or supportive and positive and contribute heavily to the formation of self-identity. Over time and through discerning awareness on the cushion, meditation works like a filter. When healing the saṃskāras of the "habit mind," it is important to sort through the internalized voices and, in particular, to dis-identify with shaming, negative voices. Through meditation, "right listening" provides a critical means to heal the schisms of a divided self.

Throat Constriction

Speaking with real truthfulness and genuine authenticity is extremely difficult. A disparity between feeling and spoken word—a translation gap—makes verbal expression challenging. Emotions are particularly difficult to express. This is exacerbated when young children are verbally shut down and told to "shut up" or "clamp it." Experiences of neglect, condemnation, fear, or repression may result in years of constriction within the throat chakra. Excessive shyness, stuttering, breathing problems, compromised listening skills, ADHD, chronic respiratory infection, and patterns of chronic immobility (freezing) may result. However, when our voice is clarified and empowered, it becomes a tremendous tool for personal growth.

There are many expressions in common parlance that identify throat constriction—gagged, choked up, made mum, tongue-tied, zipped up. When stricken by uncertainty and fear, we say that people have a "lump in the throat." Physiologically, the sides of the windpipe constrict, the vocal cords are stifled, the muscles of the neck harden, the jaw locks, and tension is held in the tongue. All of these structures are intimately connected to breathing, so in the first stages of learning to breathe mindfully we encourage students to undo the knots that bind the throat.

PRACTICE

Softening the Throat

This practice is a guide to softening the delicate structures in and around the throat. It can be done either lying in śavāsana or seated upright.

If you are lying down, be sure to support the back of your head with a folded blanket. In the seated position be sure to sit on a lift that enables you to relax your ankles and knees down to the floor. Begin by relaxing the skin of your outer face. Imagine the pores of the skin opening, as if you have just received a facial. Relax your jaw completely and allow your lips to lightly touch. Allow your tongue to rest downward behind your lower teeth. Sense your molar teeth on the upper jaw moving away from the molars on your lower jaw. By releasing mandibular restriction, your entire throat can relax.

Allow the skin around your throat and at the back of your neck to be soft, as soft as the skin of a newborn. Visualize the banks of your windpipe widening, so that your innermost throat softens. As your trachea widens imagine the topmost vertebrae of your neck, the first and second cervical vertebrae, spreading wide. Lightly tip the back of your skull upward toward the sky. Observe the texture of the breath as it brushes into your throat. See that this brush sensation is extremely light, as light as the finest hairs of a calligrapher's ink brush. Stay for five to ten minutes.

The Wind Palace

At the base of the posterior skull, where the cranium rests on top of the neck, lies a critical juncture where invasive winds can enter the body, potentially distressing the nerves. The juncture of the head and neck, as we have seen, is like a multidirectional rocking chair, and given its extensive range of motion, it is prone to bouts of distressing "wind." Where the back of the skull gains pivotal support on C1 is a key acupressure point in traditional Chinese medicine. If you palpate the bony knob in the center of the back of your skull, you are on the external occipital protruberance (EOP), the attachment site for the powerful nuchal ligament that straps the skull to the neck (see fig. 7.2). This ligament is structurally related to the mane of a horse or other grazing animal, and via its attachment to the lower cervical spine (C7-T1), provides stability for all movements of the skull. On the interior surface of the occiput (opposite to the EOP) is its sister landmark, the internal occipital protruberance. Smack in the center of the back of the skull, this interior ledge forms the attachment site for the pull of the dura, the membranous cover that wraps the spinal cord and tethers to the sacrum at the opposite end of the spine. This landmark is a critical fulcrum for craniosacral motion (see fig. 3.5).

Just below the EOP is a point traditional Chinese medicine calls the Wind Palace (DU16), named for its associations with the wind element (see figs. 2.8 and 7.2). It is part of the Governing Vessel that threads through the spinal column and enters the brain. The Governing Vessel meridian is comparable to yoga's central channel (*suṣumnā*). It serves to protect the brain and acts as a barrier to pathogens, as the high-fidelity instrument of the brain is vulnerable to disturbances of all kinds.

The Wind Palace point is used to reduce and balance any attack of the chills or respiratory colds that assail the neck. Wind invasion in traditional Chinese medicine is delightfully described as one of the "external pernicious influences," and because it is the nature of wind to penetrate any crack or crevice, it is said in the *Neijing,* a doctrinal source for traditional Chinese medicine, that "the one hundred diseases develop from the wind."[3] The neck and head are most vulnerable to wind penetration, which in turn agitates the subtle body and the entire nervous system.

When fluctuating winds invade the body, more serious conditions such as mania and fright palpitations may arise. Winds that assault the nerves disturb sleep patterns. Routine insomnia depletes the body on many levels, and in a debilitating catch-22, sleeplessness leaves one more prone to the distracting effects of wind invasion.

In yoga and Āyurveda, the nerve endings are governed by *vāta,* the wind element. We have already seen how the wind element presides over the heart, chest, and arms. When wind penetrates the neck and skull, it has corrosive effects on the nervous system. In Āyurveda aggravation of vāta leads to restlessness, excitability, and anxiety. When one is in the throes of distraction and flits from one thing to the other, we say that person is "vāta deranged."

Syndromes like ADD or ADHD, so prevalent in young children, may be attributed to a similar disturbance of the nervous system. Given the pervasiveness of the Internet and the availability of high-speed connections from laptop computers, smartphones, or mobile devices, attention ricochets from one piece of information to the next with the touch of the screen. Distraction proliferates and becomes insidious for people of all ages. Images today flick relentlessly and with such velocity that attention spans shrink and the winds of distraction are activated. Given the age of diversion we live in, the merits of concentration practice, so central to yogic training, are possibly more valuable than ever before. A pivotal part of yoga discipline, and critical for gaining access to the subtle body, is the ability to hold the attention steady in one place. In the eight limbs of Patañjali's yoga, *dhāraṇā* (focused concentration) is the sixth limb and the gateway to states of absorptive awareness. Corollary to Patañjali's Aṣṭānga Yoga, in the Noble Eightfold Path taught by the Buddha, right concentration is the last stage of the process of awakening. In the broadest sense, yogic discipline serves as an antidote to distraction, reducing the updrafts of agitation and neurotic tendency.

Vāta and Restlessness

In the traditional Buddhist framework for training the mind, five primary hindrances obstruct progress on the path. Of the five—craving, ill will, sloth, restlessness, and doubt—restlessness, related to the winds of upset, is a consequence of distraction. Whenever I teach training courses that involve investigation of the five hindrances, I ask students which hindrance is the greatest obstacle for them personally. It is interesting to note that restlessness (which includes worry) is always the most common affliction. Restlessness plagues American culture, in part due to its founding narrative, established by wayfarers who voyaged vast distances to seek a better life; and in part due to an ever-present, rapacious media bent on captivating its viewers with shorter and more sensational sound bites. A restless mind or restless heart is one that has difficulty focusing, being present, and sustaining commitment. The lightning speed of distraction upturns concentration, and as a result restlessness, agitation, and impatience may ensue—all symptoms of stormy internal winds. This is why in meditation training, we emphasize *śamatā,* for it fosters settling and deep calm in the subtle body.

Softening the Throat through Smile

When there is ease and space in the throat, there is an opportunity to expand the subtle body. This occurs by relaxing the tongue, softening the masseter muscle and internal pterygoid muscles of the jaw, and actively spreading the interior tissues of the throat. Smiling is also a valuable device for melting away frozen tension inside the throat. In Indian and Tibetan iconography, the sculpted smile carved on the beautific face of the Buddha is indicative of acceptance and nonattachment. A passage from Herman Hesse's *Siddhartha* describes the Buddha's smile this way:

> This masklike smile, this smile of unity over the flowing forms, this smile of simultaneousness over the thousands of births and deaths—this smile of Siddhartha—was exactly the same as the calm, delicate, impenetratable, perhaps gracious, perhaps mocking, wise, thousand-fold smile of Gotama, the Buddha as he perceived it with awe a hundred times. It was in such a manner, Govinda knew, that the Perfect One smiled.[4]

This thousand-fold smile suggests not only equanimity and nonclinging but a generous opening of the palate, throat, and root of the tongue. Release of the palate is suggestive of profound acceptance and an embodiment of internal knowing (*prajña*), a "wisdom beyond wisdom."

The Yoga of Sound

Another way to release constriction in the throat is through the use of sound. Just as the throat chakra is the residence of speech, it is also the source for all sound. Since time immemorial syllabic vocalization has been an instrumental way of transmitting vibration through the nāḍīs. Mantra yoga, or the yoga of sound, predates haṭha yoga and harkens back to the oral tradition of the Vedas where memorized verses evoking the mystery of the universe were chanted via a kind of prāṇāyāma. Like a classical Indian musician tuning his sitar, the subtle body can be brought into resonance through the effect of vocalized sound. The vocal cords and the larynx, along with the hollow sinus pockets within the skull, are miniature chambers for sound resonance. The subtle body vibrates as sound-wave frequencies reverberate in all tissues of the body, including the bones, glands, organs, and sinuses. Collectively, the body's physiological rhythms produce a kind of a hum, and intonating is thought to enhance acoustic resonance in the subtle body.

Sound travels in the body through fluid currents (nāḍīs), and thus the yoga of sound is called *nāda* yoga. The word *nāda* is etymologically related to the word *nāḍī*, their common root meaning to vibrate or resound. Within the subtle body the nāḍīs provide a network for sound transmission, and the syllabic sound of mantra serves to amplify vibratory rhythms throughout the body. Tonal coherence brings about greater mind-body integration and, in a more comprehensive way, harmonizes the body with *paraspanda,* the "supreme vibration" that lies at the source of all life.

PRACTICE

Throat Blossoms

This practice bestows great relaxation and ease in the throat. This exercise uses the visualization of a flower in order to dissolve constriction in the throat and create a feeling of warm effulgence in the viśuddha chakra.

Begin by sitting in a comfortable position and let go of any tension in your jaw. Soften the skin of your neck and relax your tongue, allowing it to drop as if in śavāsana. Spread the interior lining of your throat, so that the interior membranes of your windpipe become lithe and supple like the stem of a tulip. Visualize the stalk of the tulip extending down into your bronchi and lungs. Imagine the soft velvety petals of the tulip opening outward in all directions inside your throat. Imagine sublime lavender petals (the color of the throat chakra). Settle your attention along with your breath in the center of the throat flower and taste a delicate fragrance perfuming your entire throat region. Allow your breath to be softer than it has ever been before. Remain for ten minutes with this tender opening of your throat. Afterward lie down to rest for several minutes.

Celestial Sounds of the Throat

In the design of the chakras, each chakra features a resident flower with letters from the Sanskrit alphabet inscribed into each flower petal (see fig. 7.5). From the first chakra to the crown of the head, the successive chakras become more elaborate, each with a greater number of petals and more numerous syllables. Ascending through the chakras, the reverberation of letters grows more refined, and within the throat chakra the associated sounds are light and celestial. The seed sounds for each chakra (*bīja mantra*) are one-syllable mystical sounds, and by intonating each sound the "flower essence" of each chakra blooms.

The primary sound within the throat chakra is *ham,* and the peripheral bīja mantras are the sixteen Sanskrit vowels (one for each of the sixteen flower petals in the throat). The soft aspiration of *ha* in the throat expresses the delicacy and elegance of the throat and relates to the long-necked beauty of the cosmic swan, *haṃsa*. The swan or goose is revered for its ability to both swim in the earthly waters and soar into the celestial sky. Brahmā himself elects to ride the magnificent bird. The gander epitomizes the detached yogi, for the great bird swims in the earthly waters yet its feathers forever remain dry. Of all yogic mantras, the *haṃsa* refrain (and its inverse *so'ham*) is perhaps the most widely used to evoke the indivisibility of self and other. Haṃsa calls to mind the immanent and transcendent quality of the great gander, and *so'ham* is a pithy expression of the nondual (*advaita*) meaning, literally, "I am That." Like the swan that migrates through unending sky, the experience of *so'ham* involves meditative absorption into pure space.

The Primordial A *Sound*

The back of the oral cavity is the source from which the simplest of utterances is produced, such as a sigh, shriek, coo, or cry. The first sound of a newborn is a vocal emission of the out breath, a primitive guttural *a* sound. *A* is the most basic and fundamental vocalization, the origin of all speech and song. In the complex beauty of the Sanskrit language, *a* is the first letter of the Sanskrit alphabet. It is also the first letter in the Latin alphabet and in all derivitive Romance languages. In the sacred acoustics of Sanskrit, *a* stands alone as the first sound, the mother sound. It is the creator sound, the primordial source of all manifestation. It is present in all consonant letters—such as *ya, ra, la, va,* and so forth—and is the currency from which words are produced (i.e., *prāṇāyāma, ānanda,* and *Bharatanāṭyam*). *A* assumes a transcendent place in the nondual philosophy of Kashmir Śaivism. *A* is Śiva, formless yet integral to all linguistic forms. In mantra yoga, *a* is the source of power in the universe. This includes recitation of the *Aum* (Om) sound, wherein *a* is the first syllable representing creation, *u* implies maintenance, and *m* destruction. Vocalizing these three phonemes together, Aum (Om) expresses ultimate reality and the continuum from birth to death.

PRACTICE

Reciting the A *Sound*

Silently reciting *a* is a valuable way to promote width in the back of the oral cavity and generate space within the palate. This exercise enables connection with the mother sound of the Sanskrit language and the source for all becoming. This practice helps to soften the throat and relax the tongue, trachea, and vocal cords.

Begin sitting in a comfortable cross-legged position on a four- to six-inch lift so that your pelvis is above the level of your ankles. Sit in such a way that you align your skull over the middle of your chest and your chest over your pelvis. As you close your eyes, relax your jaw, the flesh of your lips, and the skin all around your throat and at the back of your neck. Then recite a soundless *a.* When you evoke the silent sound, observe the way that the membranes in your throat spread and soften. As in ujjāyī prāṇāyāma, feel the brush of the *a* sound on both the inhalation and exhalation. The mental *a* vibration should bring about a feeling of levity and connection to boundless space. Visualize the way that the mystic note *a* expands outward from the center of your throat and pervades your entire body. Remain with this visualization for five to ten minutes.

The Mandala of the Palate

The palate at the roof of the mouth is the uppermost end of the throat chakra. Anatomically, this includes a vestibule at the top of the pharynx where the cavities of the nose, mouth, and ears come together (see fig. 7.1). The nasopharynx is on the same plane as the top of the spine where the cranium rests onto the first cervical vertebra. Like a series of interlocking underground tunnels, the upper throat is where several passageways converge involving not only the sensory channels of the mouth, nose, and ears but also passageways for the respiratory, digestive, vocal, and lymphatic systems.

The palate is a thin shelf of bone that divides the oral cavity from the nasal cavity. It is part of the upper jaw and maxilla, a pneumatic bone that articulates with the spiral interior of the nasal bones. Traditional haṭha yoga texts allude to a space at the back of the throat that is a doorway directly into the subtle body. How is it that the alcove at the back of the soft palate, set within the cavern of the mouth, is held in such high regard? Descriptions of this area are steeped in cryptic language and mythological reference and thus are difficult to decipher.

The palate has reciprocity with the perineum as neurological reflexes relay between the oral cavity and the pelvic cavity. Freud mapped the significance of the oral and anal stages of neurological development in the first three years of life. Psychological issues pertaining to nurturing, intimacy, control, and libidinal drive are linked to these two erogenous zones. Coincidentally, the primary pathway of the vital kuṇḍalinī is from perineum to palate.

The palate is called the *talumaṇḍalam* in Sanskrit (*talu* simply means surface), and like the soles of the feet, we could think of it as another interior map to the subtle body. In Hindu and Buddhist art, a *maṇḍala* is a design made up of thresholds within thresholds, a kind of microcosm of the universe used by meditators to navigate the interior labyrinth of the mind.

The maṇḍala of the palate is akin to a vaulted interior dome that divides the sacred world from the profane. In sacred architecture vaulted domes are thresholds to celestial realms. The semispheric ceiling of a mosque or the vaulted ceiling of a fourteenth-century cathedral are examples. Similarly, in the kiva design of the Pueblo people in the Southwestern United States, an uppermost hatchway door leads to the subterranean ceremonial space. The antechamber of the oral cavity is reminiscent of the kind of cave told in the Native American myth of origination (recounted at the beginning of this book). It is a portal leading to physical and spiritual birth. In the architecture of the human body, the palate, along with the cranial base, is the uppermost threshold that leads to the firmament of the skull.

The Palate and the Path of the Suṣumnā

The palate is comprised of two paired bones, with a fissure or seam down the middle. You can feel this seam by placing the tip of your tongue on the roof of your mouth. This seam coincides with the zigzag suture at the very crown of the head (sagittal suture) that divides the right and left half of the skull. It is significant that these two bony seams mirror each another. Centered on the body's median axis, they are thought to be throughways for the passage of the sublime central channel.

I imagine that if it were at all in their power to do so, haṭha yogis would directly enter the cranium in order to monitor brain activity and produce a selfless, more illumined consciousness. However, the orb of the skull is strategically sealed in order to safeguard the vital organ of the brain. In lieu of direct access, yogis curl the tip of their tongue backward and press it against the roof of the mouth or slide it even farther, into the soft pocket at the back of the nasopharynx (see fig. 7.1). Given the palate's proximity to the brain, this movement is thought to monitor brain activity. Retracting the tongue and inserting it into the vestibule behind the soft palate is called *khechari mudrā.* This is meant to seal the gap where the precious ambrosia flows down and preserve the deep life-force:

> The channel called *Suṣumnā,* serving as a passage for the *prāṇa,* cuts through the palate. When there is *yoga* of the breath, the mind and *Aum,* then the *prāṇa* goes upward. By revolving the tip of the tongue back on the palate and yoking the senses, let

> greatness perceive greatness. Then one reaches selflessness. Because one is selfless, one no longer experiences *sukha* or *dukha.* For thus has it been said, "Having stabilized the *prāṇa*, that has been restrained, having crossed the barrier, one is yoked to the unlimited at the crown of the head."[5]

The vestibule at the back of the oral cavity is partially veiled by a teardrop-shaped piece of flesh called the uvula that dangles from the roof of the mouth. If you have never identified your uvula, the next time you look in the bathroom mirror, open your mouth wide as you would in *simhāsana* (lion pose) and you will see a soft structure suspended from the back of your palate. This flap, along with the tonsils that are tucked behind it, functions as part of the immune system. When swallowing, the soft palate and the uvula pull upward to seal off the nasal cavity so that food or liquid does not enter.

In the esoteric anatomy of the yogic system, the uvula, like a stalactite suspended from the roof of a cave, is where drops of nectar are purported to drip out of the skull into the throat. The notion of a divine serum or sacred drink of the gods, whose source is an interior font within the skull, appears prominently in the esoteric manuals on yoga. Physiologically, these droplets of immortality (*amṛta*) may in fact be hormonal distillations secreted from the pituitary gland, the master gland within the skull located just millimeters above the top of the nasopharynx (see fig. 7.1). We have seen how the chakras reflect the glandular centers in the body and the powerful sway that hormones have over biological function. By inserting the tongue into the vestibule behind and above the soft palate, the yogi sought to monitor secretions from this most influential gland.

PRACTICE

Jihva Mudrā: The Tongue Seal

This meditation is a version of a centuries-old technique involving turning the tongue backward in the mouth. It serves to broaden the palate and release strain at the back of the throat.

Begin by sitting comfortably so that your spine and pelvis are supported. Sit on a four- to six-inch cushion so that there is lift and lightness in your sacral area. When sitting, gently raise the back of your skull up toward the ceiling and descend your jaw slightly downward. Relax your mandible by wiggling your jaw side to side and then allow your jaw to slide down away from your ears. Then curl the tip of your tongue upward and rest it behind your upper front two teeth. This is the initial position for the tongue. Feel the way your lower jaw begins to relax further downward. Then slide your tongue back to the very center of your palate. Lightly push upward against the midline of the roof of your mouth with your tongue tip. Imagine that you are opening a small parasol inside your mouth. Feel your palate spread as you create space between your lower and upper teeth. Consequently sense your entire cranial base spreading horizontally.

Remain with a very light pressure (as much pressure as you would use when raising a dimmer on a light switch) for five to ten minutes. This inner seal can be done at any time, while driving, listening to music, or when you're in āsana. It is the seed movement for khechari mudrā, which involves turning the tongue all the way back behind the soft palate.

The Convergence of Three Rivers

In the ancient religious traditions of India, the conjunction of three rivers is considered a most holy place. The site of the Kumbha Mela, the world's largest pilgrimage where up to 80 million Hindus gather every twelve years in Allahabad, north India, is where three rivers converge—the Ganga, the Yamuna, and the mythical underground Saraswati River. Here devotees come to bathe, cleanse, purify, and make ritual offerings. The site of the Kumbha Mela is considered sacred because it is believed that droplets of the immortal soma fell from the sky from a pot carried by the gods following the churning of the Ocean of Milk.

In the geography of India it is thought that the "body" of the land bears likeness to the organization of the physical body. In the topography of the subtle body, the throat is the confluence of three rivers—the auditory tubes, the nasal cavity, and the oral cavity. Like the site of the sacred ground of the Kumbha Mela, the back of the throat is where three great rivers that convey prāṇa in the subtle body—the idā, piṇgalā, and suṣumnā nāḍīs—converge. It is here in the contours of the throat that droplets of a divine nectarine liquid are reputed to "fall from the heaven" of the skull.

Drops of Divine Nectar and Blue Throat

One of the best-known and well-loved myths of India tells of the trial to capture and retain these precious drops of nectar within the throat plexus. This tale involves the struggle between malevolent and divine forces and of precarious thresholds involving the pure and the toxic. The story, "The Churning of the Ocean of Milk," begins with the primordial ocean at the beginning of time and ends in Śiva's throat, revealing a fluid potency in both realms. We saw in chapter 2 how the tale describes reptilian forces relating to kuṇḍalinī. The *kūrma* (the turtle) is stationed at the bottom of the ocean (as part of the first chakra) in order to support Mount Meru, the first global landmass, on its back. When the gods and demons performed their ontological tug-of-war, pulling at opposite ends of the cosmic serpent (*ādiśeṣa*), the earth mass was set in motion. At the ocean surface rotational forces caused the waters to churn, and from this blender-like turning (*vṛtti*), all of life emerged.

The competitive roil between the two forces—one benevolent, the other ruinous—was an all-out pursuit of the immortal nectar (amṛta) hidden in the mountain/spine. Thus, gods and demons enacted the first tapas, and the agitated whir of the ocean revealed the supreme life-sustaining substance called *soma*. The creation myth implies the procreative act and the friction necessary to produce life. When the writhing was over, however, a black and toxic substance emerged, one that was impossible for either the gods or the demonic forces to handle. So they beamed a satellite call to Śiva, for who but Śiva, the harbinger of both creation and death, had the capacity to cope with such a poison? Śiva summarily drank the toxic film yet, due to his yogic powers of sorcery and the unlimited power of his tapas, did not swallow it. Rather, via jālandhara bandha he caught the poison in his throat so it did not seep down, metastasize, and destroy his body. The substance underwent an alchemical conversion, and Śiva's neck turned a deep ocean blue, the color of a brilliant sapphire. From that day on, Śiva was referred to as *Nīlakaṇṭha* (Blue Throat), and his azure skin proved to be alluring to the ladies. In fact Parvati, Śiva's divine consort, confessed that it was the radiance of the skin on Śiva's neck that enticed her into his arms.

Śiva's power of transmutation and decontamination, converting poison into passion and intoxication into purity, is related to the alchemical process of kuṇḍalinī yoga. Śiva's power to disinfect relates to the protective role of the immune system, guarding the body against impurities especially in and around the throat. The story of the Blue Throat god suggests the potency associated with the throat, a potency linked not only to immunological health and the refinement and purification of prāṇa but also to the cultivation of yogic power.

Within the esoteric yoga tradition, purification of the throat region leads to an accumulation of astonishing powers. For example, in the Yoga Sutras of Patañjali in the chapter on extraordinary accomplishments (*vibhūti*), it is said that through profound meditation on the "throat well" the yogi overcomes craving of all kinds (*kaṇṭha kūpe kṣut pipāsā nivṛttiḥ* III.30). Nonattachment is identified in classical yoga as "going beyond cravings of hunger and thirst," signifying that the practitioner, having attained the highest state of being, need not ingest or experience anything else.

In the next chapter, we will see how the space within the cranial vault is heralded to be the source for the highest wisdom and the experience of samādhi. In this chapter we have seen how the throat, and particularly the palate, is a direct and expedient means to access the subtle body. Now we enter the interior of the cranium itself, a move that requires exquisite delicacy and yet is the culmination of the journey through the chakras.

8

THE CROWN JEWEL

Light on Infinite Space

This mind through endless kalpas without beginning, has never varied. It has never lived or died, appeared or disappeared, increased or decreased. It's not pure or impure, good or evil, past or future. It's not true or false. It's not male or female. . . . It strives for no realization and suffers no karma. It has no strength or form. It's like space, you can't possess it and you can't lose it. Its movements can't be blocked by mountains, rivers or rock walls.

—From *The Zen Teachings of Bodhidharma*, "Bloodstream Sermon"[1]

Releasing tension within the skull is a critical part of yoga training, for only by unlocking the structures in and around the brain, packed with billions of neurons, can a sense of ease pervade the entire nervous system. Yoga practice emphasizes pacification of all the structures within the skull—the cranial bones, the cranial muscles, and, most important, the sensory organs. Without relaxation of these exquisitely fine tissues, it is difficult for the brain to rest in profound states of meditation (samādhi). Thus, haṭha yoga underscores the importance of pratyāhāra—softening and sublimating sensory awareness.

Much like a medieval palace, the body only permits entry through its primary gates. The input and outflow of sensory stimuli is thought to pass through nine "gates," seven of which are in the cranium: the two eyes, two nostrils, two ears, and the mouth. In the way that sentries protect the palace gates, yogis safeguard these thresholds. Closing the ears, turning the tongue tip against the roof of the mouth, and fixing the eyes to the midline help monitor the flow of activity through the sensory gates. The two other apertures reside in the pelvic floor, and mūla bandha presides over these lower gates.

By internalizing the senses, the yogi reunites with the source of prāṇa within him. In the Bhagavad Gītā, when Arjuna asks Kṛṣṇa what the greatest of all sacrifices is, Kṛṣṇa responds:

> By sealing off the gates of the body and
> absorbing the mind in the heart,
> concentrating the vital breath (prāṇa) in the cranium,
> one becomes established in meditation.[2]

We saw earlier how the turtle is prized in yoga for its capacity to withdraw its limbs (see fig. 2.7). This retraction and ensuing interiority is an analogy for pratyāhāra. On the path of yoga, turning the mind inward upon itself, away from the peripheral gates, reveals its empty and clear nature. In the successive path of Patañjali's eight limbs of yoga, pratyāhāra follows āsana and prāṇāyāma and is a necessary prelude to the last three meditative limbs—*dhāraṇā, dhyāna,* and *samādhi.* In Aṣṭāṅga Yoga, the first four limbs—*yama, niyama, āsana,* and *prāṇāyāma*—are referred to as the outer limbs (*bahiraṅga*), and the last four, beginning with pratyāhāra, are identified as the inner limbs (*antaraṅga*). Profound involution on the path of yoga illuminates the subtle body. Monitoring the flow of stimuli through the sensory gates not only mitigates intracranial stress, what one of my teachers described as "brain squeeze," but also promotes delicate shifts within the brain's neurochemistry.

We could say that of all the organs in the body, the brain is the most difficult to affect or change; it cannot be physically adjusted. We can manipulate the large intestine, liver, or stomach by flexing or extending the spine, and it is possible to alter the rhythmic contractions of the heart and lungs via regulated breathing. But it is impossible to manipulate the brain, which is carefully enshrined in the orb of the cranial vault. Thus, states of meditation, heart-centered loving-kindness (metta), and the vibratory rhythms of mantra vicariously influence command centers deep within the brain.

In the meditative traditions, absorption into the innermost sublime channel of the body produces profound neurological and hormonal shifts. Diminished tension within the skull (and the entire nervous system) fosters ease in the sensitive tissues of the brain, including the brain stem, cranial nerves, endocrine glands, and spinal cord. When tension lessens, respiratory rhythms slow, the long tide of the cranial rhythm sets in, heart rate decreases, and the regulatory activity of the parasympathetic nerves increases. In the wisdom teachings, these shifts involve a reorganization of the psyche away from the view of a solid, independent self. This shift affords a kind of transparency where a divided, dualistic frame of mind erodes and an all-pervasive awareness stands as the source for each sensory and psychic experience.

Before we continue our journey to the top of the skull and explore the profound energetics of the brain, we need to examine some of the structures involved in sensory awareness. First we will investigate the jaw, as tensions within the jaw have a pervasive effect on the cranium and entire body. Then we will explore the ear and the importance of the ear to the flow of prāṇa. Finally we will see how the gates of the eyes play a dominant role in sensory perception. Balancing the intricate structures that contain the sensory organs is critical to cranial mechanics and the fluid dynamics of the brain.

The Maw of the Jaw

In an ideal posture, there is no muscular tension held above the collarbones; that is, the neck, jaw, and skull are free of mechanical stress. Unfortunately, structural and psychological tension tends to burrow into the structures surrounding the brain, including the connective tissues of the scalp, the cranial bones, the facial muscles, and the jaw. When pressure mounts in the body, the powerful muscles that attach the jaw to the skull clench. When the jaw grips, it is part of the body's protective mechanism to safeguard the vital structures of the brain and throat.

What makes the cranium so unusual—and difficult to work with—is that the upper skull consists of bones that are relatively fixed, whereas the lower skull includes the highly mobile jawbone (fig 8.1). Twenty-two bones comprise the skull and face, and only one of them—the mandible—moves freely. The mandible can articulate in numerous directions, it can move sideways, protract forward, retract backward, and rotate. The function of the jaw is complex. It is a multitasker, performing a multitude of roles in the body relating to digestion, respiration, and immunity. As part of the apparatus that generates speech, it is involved in verbal articulation. It is a structure that exhibits emotion: muscular tension in the jaw conveys feelings that range from intimacy and love to fear and disgust. We have all experienced a tightly knitted jaw in moments of anger and self-defense, a slack jaw when relaxed and sleepy, or a soft, wide, and open jaw in moments of laughter and fun. In short, the mandible encapsulates the self as internal feeling states confer readily to the jaw.

The mandible's proximity to the brain and sensory organs is a structural predicament, for the jaw is a veritable magnet for emotional and psychological tension. This has pervasive effects on brain function, as 38 percent of the neurological input to the brain comes from the nerves that innervate the face, mouth, and temporal mandibular joint (TMJ).[3]

For adults and an increasing number of children, muscular tension in the jaw causes the TMJ to misalign. When the jaw does not track symmetrically, it can distress the delicate architecture of the skull.

Figure 8.1 The Temporal Mandibular Joint

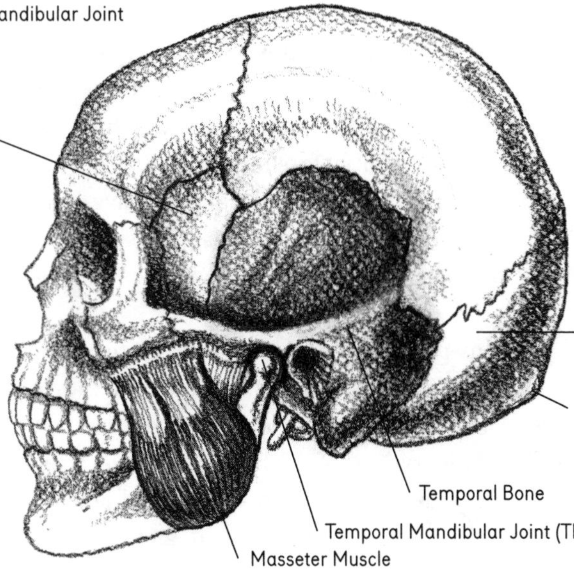

Daily psychological pressures involving money, family demands, and work readily contribute to temporal mandibular strain.

Along with the solar plexus that we reviewed in chapter 3, the jaw is invested with the power of will. When our will is thwarted or repressed, it is common for the jaw to clench and stiffen. Ambition, competitiveness, and resolve show up as the jutting, locked jaw look of John Wayne. Like a clenched fist, held anger, trapped rage, and repressed grief manifest as a tight jaw. The jaw bears the brunt of emotional pain that stems from lack of love, protection, or intimacy. However, laughter and smiling are the body's way of expressing joy, delight, and love and serve to relax the powerful musculature of the jaw.

In the face of life-threatening situations, both real and imagined, the jaw is one of the first bodily structures to constrict. In chapter 5, we reviewed the consequence of what Thomas Hanna, in his book *Somatics,* coined the "red-light reflex." Here, he describes what happens to the jaw at the outset of that reflex:

> If a woman walking down a street hears the sudden explosion of a car backfiring, this is what happens: Within 14 milliseconds the muscles of her jaw begin to contract; this is immediately followed about 20 milliseconds later by a contraction of her eyes and brow. But before her eyes have squeezed shut, her shoulder and neck muscles (the trapezius) have received a neural impulse at 25 milliseconds to contract, raising her shoulders and bringing her head forward.[4]

This protective response contributes to both anterior drag of the shoulder (see fig. 6.5) and kyphotic curvature in the upper back (see fig. 7.4). It is a primitive neuromuscular reflex, tied to centers deep in the limbic system of the brain that govern self-defense. Trapped pain in the body may result in a hardened jaw; however, when the body-mind is suddenly overwhelmed, as in a surprise attack, the jaw may go limp and fall. In instances of great loss, defeat, sadness, or the point of surrender, the jaw lets go in what is colloquially called a "jaw-dropping" experience.

When under stress, the jaw binds to the temporal bones with which it articulates (thus the name temporal mandibular joint). This is due primarily to the powerful masseter muscle that holds the mandible to the skull. You can palpate the ropy fibers of the masseter just below your outer cheek bones. The TMJ joint is shaped like a ball-and-socket joint (although it it classified as a hinge-and-sliding joint), and in the dynamics of the subtle body, its location on the lateral sides of the skull correlates to the ball-and-socket joint on the lateral side of the pelvis. In structural dynamics of the pelvis and skull, reciprocal tension is held in both the mandibular joints and the hip joints.

The Jaws of Life or Death

In the animal kingdom, the jaw harbors an ancient reflex wired toward survival. Under threat, animals bare their teeth, chomp their jaws, and snarl. Part throat and part cranium, the jaw is an ancient structure designed not only to trap and ingest food but also to protect and defend. It is a most ancient and incisive tool that effectively determines whether one eats or is eaten. Over millions of years of evolution, dating back to the eras of T. rex and the saber-toothed tiger, the jaw is the quintessential bone in the body that is called to action in a life-or-death response. Through innumerable fight-to-the-finish challenges, animals attack and defend with the powerful clamping reflex of the jaw. The human mandible retains this prehistoric reflex.

PRACTICE

Releasing the Jaw

This practice is a valuable way to dissolve tension held in the mandible. It can be done at work, while waiting in traffic, or right before you fall asleep at night. Practice on your back in śavāsana, so that gravitational forces that impact the neck and skull are released.

Lie with your head supported by a two-inch blanket lift. Exhale deeply a few times in order to deflate any tension that may be buried in your jaw. Allow your tongue to drop to the floor of your mouth behind your lower teeth. Practice śavāsana in your jaw—that is, release the skin below your ears, at the center of your chin, and above your upper lip. Allow your jaw to go a bit slack, so that your mandible drops away from your upper jaw. Notice your back molars, and be sure that your upper and lower teeth move away from each other. Allow your lips to part ever so slightly. Continue to do śavāsana in your tongue so that it drops and spreads wide like a banana leaf. Now open your mouth about 30 degrees and place the heel of your hand against the center of your chin (on the lowermost portion of the mandible called the mental protruberance). Open your jaw by extending your mandible forward while at the same time resisting the protraction of your jaw with the heel of your hand. Continue to open your jaw by degrees while continuing to provide resistance. As you open incrementally, you will be stretching different fibers of your masseter muscles, pterygoid muscles, and the TMJ ligaments that hold the mandible in place. Then place the heel of your hand on the side of your jaw, and with your jaw open, move your jaw to the side, once more against resistance. Again open by degrees and continue to push and resist. This stretches the opposite masseter and pterygoid muscles. Repeat on the other side.

Do the entire exercise for five minutes. Then close your jaw and notice any heat or strain dissipate from your face, TMJs, and ears. Allow a feeling of lightness and softness to pervade your entire skull.

Space and the Divine Ear

The temporal bones are beautiful fan-shaped bones whose bony matrix houses the orifice of the ear. The ear has three distinct compartments. The duct of the outer ear leads to a mini-diaphragm, the tympanic membrane. The vestibule of the middle ear is filled with space and is continuous with the uppermost part of the throat via the auditory tubes (figs. 7.1 and 8.2). The ear houses miniature bones that tap signals to the brain like Morse code. The malleus (hammer) taps the incus (the anvil), which taps the stapes (the stirrup). The stapes, the smallest bone in the body, transmits sound into the inner ear. The inner ear houses a spiral seashell-like structure, the cochlea (Greek for conch shell), that emits sound signals directly to the brain by way of the vestibulocochlear nerve. The inner ear is filled with fluid where

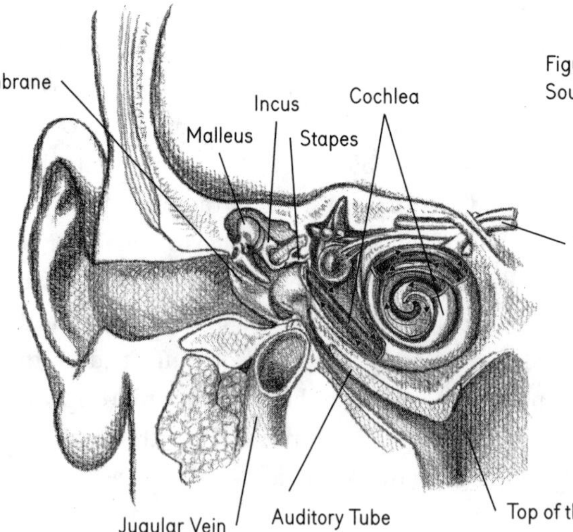

Figure 8.2 The Pathway of Sound through the Inner Ear

thousands of specialized hair cells register postural changes within the body's connective tissues and joints.

The refined and delicate apparatus of the ear stands in sharp contrast to the powerful, strapping structures of the mandible positioned just millimeters away. Compression of the TMJ causes the mandible to pin upward against the temporal bones, potentially inhibiting their motion and compromising the diminutive bones of the inner ear. The rigors involved in chewing—grinding, tugs, trauma to the teeth—frequently cause bruxism (teeth grinding) and affect the delicate equilibrium of the temporal bones. When the TMJ is free of restrictions the entire skull can decompress and feelings of ease and serenity spread through the cranium.

In meditation practices, it is valuable to mindfully "float" the temporal bones to induce calm and relaxation within the brain. This may have vicarious effects on the temporal lobes of the brain that contour to the interior concave surface of the temporal bone. The temporal lobes process auditory input, organize language and speech, and store memory.

Of all the sensory organs, the ears provide the most immediate and extensive connection to the subtle body. Not only do the ears link to the interior breath and the flow of prāna but they are gateways to the entire audible realm, considered to be sacred in yoga. More so than the eyes, the ears are portals to the subtle body. Unlike the visual field wherein visual images leave lasting impressions on the brain, sound is ephemeral and its imprints are harder to trace. The ears provide direct connection to the transitoriness of the world, whereas visual impressions make the things of the world *seem* permanent and real.

All sound travels through the atmosphere and thus the ear is identified with *ākāśa* (space). Ākāśa is the fifth and most refined of the five elements (see fig. 1.1). *Ākāśa* in Sanskrit refers to that which is indivisible; it is suggestive of pure space—that which cannot be divided, deconstructed, or reduced in any way. In order to conceptualize the ethereal realm of ākāśa, one might imagine the summit of any of the lofty Himalayan peaks where the air thins and atmospheric pressure decreases. Śiva resides at the zenith of the Himalayas at an altitude where air (vāta) turns to space (ākāśa). Similarly, in the topography of the body the etheric element resides in the summit of the cranium.

Space is the substratum from which all the other material elements emerge; prāṇa too is born of space. The importance of the space and its affiliate connection to the ear is explained in the third chapter of the Patañjali's Yoga Sutras on *siddhis* (extraordinary powers). It is said that through deep listening the ear dissolves into pure space and we gain a "divine ear" (*śrotra ākāśayoḥ saṃbandha saṃyamād divyaṃ śrotraṃ,* III.41). A divine ear is one that awakens to pure consciousness via sound. As we saw in chapter 7, sound and syllabic resonance enliven the subtle body as they vibrate through the nāḍīs. Mantras' reverberating effects purify the body's subtle channels. Similarly, in ujjāyī prāṇāyāma, the ear attunes to the whisper of breath, wherein a sibilant sound is just audible to the inner ear. In the subtle body, the inner ear fosters connection to divine sound called *śabda Brāhma*, literally "sound of the creator." Thus, sound transmission brings about affinity with the innermost spirit.

In our journey from the base of the body to the crown of the head, we have migrated from the solid ground of earth in the feet to the realm of space that resides in the sanctuary of the skull. In the wisdom traditions, space together with the mind are considered to be all-pervasive. The element of space in the meditative traditions cannot be overemphasized, although at the same time, it is not really an element, given that it is immaterial and has no characteristic or trait. Ākāśa or space is likened to emptiness. Space not only is linked to the ear but also has domain over the crown chakra. *Sahasrāra* (the crown chakra), known as the 1,000-petaled lotus, is also referred to as the empty chakra (*śūnya chakra*). Thus, an enlightened mind is equated with boundless space and is imagined to be like pure sky. Śiva resides at the top of the spinal edifice, and is referred to as the one who is "made of sky" or is made of "sacred space" (*vyoman deva*).

The cranial chakras are akin to the upper stratosphere of the sky that spreads like a cover over the world. Through intuitive realization yogis perceived that the microcosm of the body is equated with the macrocosm of the universe. In this light, the cranium has the quality of a celestial, heavenly sphere. Space is not limited to the celestial realm; rather, space pervades everything from the smallest atomic particle to the outermost galaxy. Space is equated with pure consciousness and, like space, consciousness is boundless. This all-pervasive nature of space is celebrated by the Tibetan hermit-mystic Shabkar, living in the late 1700s on retreat high in the Himalayan plateau:

> By virtue of its all penetrating freedom,
> This total presence has no center or circumference,
> No inside or outside,
> Is innocent of all partiality and
> Knows no blocks or barriers.
> This all penetrating intrinsic awareness
> Is a vast expanse of space.
> All experience of samsāra and nirvāṇa
> Arise in it like rainbows in the sky.[5]

Space Time and Inner-Ear Equilibrium

While the ear is associated with space, it is interesting to note that the temporal bone that houses the opening to the ear is associated with time. The word *temporal* stems from the Latin word *tempus*, meaning time. The temporal bone was so named because it is where hair first grays, demonstrating the trajectory of time. Time and space are part of an inseparable continuum as Albert Einstein declared in the beginning of the twentieth century. The objective of yogic discipline for millennia has been to recognize that time is an illusion contingent upon perspective and that it is not fixed or absolute. Space is also not absolute, because space only takes on identity relative to substance. Yogis have sought to move beyond the limitations of linear time and space, and so the meditative, sacrosanct ears are openings into an "all-penetrating intrinsic awareness."

Yoga poses and the flowing movements of tai chi or qigong are means to train the inner ear. The ear governs balance, and every shift in posture (including simple movements such as standing up after a nap on the couch), involves pressure changes within the inner ear. Poses such as *parivṛtta trikonāsana* (revolved triangle), headstand, or backbends require minute and subtle calibrations within the inner ear. By extending to the periphery of one's hands or feet in downward-facing dog pose or by balancing on one leg in the half moon pose, one develops greater inner equilibrium, spatial awareness, and proprioceptive awareness.

Education of the Inner Ear

Vestibular training of the inner ear benefits young children as they grow. My son attends a Waldorf School that follows the Rudolph Steiner methodology of education. Between the ages of five to seven, a child is taught somatic awareness and vestibular equilibrium by walking on low-to-the-ground balance beams, standing on short stilts, and balancing on one leg. In this way, the Steiner schools aim to advance kinesthetic intelligence prior to cognitive development. Spatial orientation and kinesthetic awareness help train a child's proprioception as the brain develops. This serves to support and ground a child's intellectual growth, thus assuring overall embodiment of learning. Education of the inner ear may be of particular benefit for children who frequently struggle with issues regarding personal boundaries, attention span, and physical confidence.

Listening and inner-ear development begin in utero. In fetal development, the ear begins to register the cacophony of sounds produced by the mother. In utero, a growing fetus adapts to her mother's respiratory rhythm and absorbs her "breath print." If you have ever had the opportunity to listen to a sonogram recording of the soft thump of a fetal heartbeat, you may recall hearing the gurgle, slosh, and murmur of the mother's digestive and circulatory flow. In utero, a growing fetus absorbs all the ambient sounds of the mother. Studies have shown that during embryonic development, little beings can respond to acoustic stimuli both from within the mother and from outside sources. The auditory capacity of a fetus suggests that the ear is one of the first sensory organs to develop (along with the lips and tongue that develop during fetal thumb sucking). This notion of the ear as an early sensory organ runs parallel to the ancient Vedic belief that the ear fosters connection to primordial sound.

In the yoga tradition, the beautiful contours of the inner ear are likened to a conch shell (fig. 8.2). In fact the temporal bone that houses the orifice of the ear is called the conch bone in Sanskrit (*śaṅkha asthi*). The conch in the yoga tradition signifies pure sound. Throughout the history of India, it has been considered a divine instrument, as it beckons devotees to prayer in spiritual communities. Also, its piercing blast historically signaled a call to action on the battlefield, and its blare heralds the beginning of battle in the Bhagavad Gītā. The trumpeting conch transmits clear, penetrating sound and its peal is used to enliven and wake up the nāḍīs. Throughout Buddhist and Hindu iconography, avatars and deities are depicted holding a conch. Patañjali is depicted holding a conch, a wheel, and a sword (*śaṅkha-chakra-asi*): the conch suggesting divine sound, the wheel the spin of time, and the sword discriminating awareness.

PRACTICE

The Conch Mudrā

The sensorimotor nerve pathways that enervate the fingers and thumbs occupy significant areas of the brain. In this practice you will learn the hand movement for *śaṅkha mudrā* (the conch mudrā) that correlates to the pathway of sound in the innermost ear.

Begin by sitting comfortably on a four- to six-inch lift. Sit with an upright spine and balance your skull so that the miniature seashells of your ears are poised within the temporal bones. Bring sensitivity to the movement of air as it wafts into your ear. Relax your jaw and tongue and visualize your cheekbones lifting and widening. After several minutes of śamatā (establishing an open and relaxed awareness), raise your hands in front of your chest. Extend your left hand vertically upward as if you are doing the *namaste* gesture with one hand. Then clasp your left thumb in your right palm. Then lay your left fingers over the back of your right hand. While doing so bring your right thumb together with the pads of your left index, middle, and ring fingers. Observe the shape of your mudrā. It should resemble the overlapping spirals of a conch shell. Set the hand position in front of your chest, then close your eyes and bring your awareness to the sonorous rhythm of your breath. Make the sound of your breath like the sound of a distant ocean, similar to what you hear when you place your ear to the opening in a conch shell. Connect to the primordial sound of the ocean through the echo of your own prāṇa. Remain for ten minutes, then relax in śavāsana at the end.

Listening with the Third Ear

In meditation, it is valuable to soften the muscular attachments around the jaw in order to release the delicate inner ear and connect to interior silence. Yoking to silence imparts a soothing effect on the entire brain while promoting śamatā—profound ease and serenity throughout the body. This meditation serves to bring stillness and space within the skull by imagining a third ear (like the mystical third eye) in the center skull.

Sit in a comfortable position and align your skull on top of your spinal column in such a way that the back of your skull floats upward and your temporal bones widen away from each other. Listen to the movement of the wind of your breath as it brushes against your nostrils and throat and into the lungs. Relax the weight of your jaw downward in order to decompress your temporal mandibular joints. Soften all the skin around your ears. Imagine your earlobes draping downward, like those of the Buddha (long earlobes are a sign of wisdom in yoga training). Soften the skin that leads into the ear canal (external auditory meatus) and into your eardrum (tympanic membrane). Sense a fluid equilibrium within your inner ears.

Balance your skull so that you feel a sense of harmony between your right and left ears. With the feeling of serenity in your outer ears, bring your awareness inside your skull to a point midway between your two anatomical ears. Visualize a third ear at the top of your brain stem. At this point, your visualization might replicate the spiral shape of an actual ear or you may imagine an open cavity in your mid-skull that absorbs sound. As you listen with this third mystical ear avoid trying to identify the sounds you hear. Do not grasp at the sound or attempt to make sense of the sound; rather, practice unfiltered, pure listening. Notice your connection to sound and observe your connection to silence. Continue to soften your anatomical ears, as you become absorbed by your imagined third ear. As you listen, bring the tip of your tongue to the roof of your mouth to widen the back of your palate and soften the entry to your windpipe. Stay for ten minutes or more breathing with a light ujjāyī breath. Rest afterward in śavāsana.

Humming Like a Bee

In the way that children hum to themselves to soothe their biorhythms, this practice fosters a soothing resonance inside the skull and throughout the spinal nerves. This technique involves closing off the entryway to the ears and directing the mind to the murmur of breath. Called *bhrāmari prāṇāyāma* (the bumblebee breath) for the way the inner drone resembles that of a humming bee, the overall effect is absorbing.

Begin by lying on your back with a bolster under your knees and your head supported by a blanket. If you have two blocks, place the blocks on either side of your skull near your ears. Rest in śavāsana for several minutes and attune to the rhythm of your breath as you did in the "Sensing the Breath Print" exercise in chapter 6. Once your breath settles into a smooth and relaxed rhythm, then close the entry to each ear by inserting the pads of your index fingers into the opening of your two ear canals. Alternatively, you can push the tragus, or frontal ear flap, over the entrance to your ear. Prop your elbows onto the blocks so that there is no strain or gripping in your shoulders. Observe the interior resonance of your breath. It should sound like you are breathing underwater from a scuba diving tank. Listen to the sonorous rhythm of your inner breath while doing the ujjāyī prāṇāyāma. Observe the pitch and purr of your breath. Then on the exhalation, generate a low humming sound. This is called *brāhmari prāṇāyāma,* and the sound mimics a bumblebee inside a flower. The vibration of the inner drone should reverberate through your entire skull. You can alter the pitch of your hum, yet the lower pitches tend to foster greater relaxation. Continue for five minutes. Then slowly lower your arms and observe as a soothing and spacious feeling pervades your entire body.

Inner Vision

In subtle body training, while a capacity for listening is heightened, dominance of the visual field is diminished. In the way that the ears are associated with space, the eyes are identified with form. Form is associated with desire that tantalizes and distracts, tricking the mind into believing its own mirrored images are real.

Fluctuation within the eye contributes to the production of thought patterns in the forebrain, like the way rapid eye movements (REM) flicker across the screen of the mind in sleep. As the eyes flutter and dance they prompt a narrative of images. In waking, when the eyes dart rapidly to and fro, they indicate restlessness, distraction, or heightened levels of activation. From an early time, yogis sensed that an extensive portion of the brain is devoted to the visual field and that seeing is a form of sensory reasoning. To temporarily arrest the reason-making function within the brain, the yogi holds his eyes steady (*trataka*).

Relaxing the eyes fosters a parasympathetic response in the body. Haṭha yoga requires fixing the gaze (*dṛṣṭi*) on various points of the body such as the tip of the finger, the nose, or the heart. When I learned vinyāsa yoga from Pattabhi Jois in Mysore in 1989, the alchemy of the practice involved four primary components: movement, breathing, bandha, and dṛṣṭi. Stilling the gaze is a very old yogic method. For example, concentrating the eyes at the centerpoint (*bindu*) of the Sri Yantra detailed in chapter 3 (see fig. 3.6) is meant to make the mind one-pointed (*ekāgrata).*

It is interesting to note that in much of the world today, people fix their eyes on a small screen for hours on end. Locking your eyes onto a computer screen has a very different effect than the yoga method dṛṣṭi, designed to slow the synaptic firings of the neocortex. When you focus your eyes on a screen, they vacillate here and there, stimulating the visual cortex of the brain. Many young children spend long periods of time with their eyes glued to a small screen during their formative years. Restricting the eyes to a computer screen may adversely affect the overall neuroplasticity of the brain.

While yogis pacify their anatomical eyes there is a corollary opening of a mystical eye, associated not with outer seeing but with inner seeing. Śiva is known as the "Three-Eyed One" (*tryambakaṃ*), and inner vision (*antara dṛṣṭi*) lies at the heart of spiritual development. In meditation, wisdom is derived from insight (*vipassana*) into the mind's empty nature.

In the Yoga Sutras it is said that when oscillating patterns of distraction subside, the eye of inner wisdom is unobstructed and the timeless Seer "stands in its own essential form," *tadā draṣṭuḥ svarūpe avasthānam* (I.3). The analogy of the Seer or interior witness is used to describe pure awareness. Pure awareness is not something gained or lost, activated or made passive. Rather it is unchanging and incorruptible. There are many referents for it, including Śiva, buddha nature, unconditioned mind, and naked awareness. The label is not so important. Rather the yogi's prerogative is to directly experience and "see into" the essential luminosity of mind.

The Sphenoid and the Body of Light

The eye of wisdom, or third eye as it is often referred to, is located along the body's central axis, at the center brow. The mystical eye of wisdom is signified by a bindu in the middle of the forehead worn by Hindus for both adornment and religious purposes. This focal point, just above the bridge of the nose, is the hub of the sixth chakra, the ājñā chakra. This point refers to the interior of the brain. If we imagine a cross section through the brain and skull at the level of the midbrow, then the third-eye center is associated with a cluster of structures around the brain stem including the hypothalamus, pituitary, and pineal glands (fig. 8.3). The hypothalamus oversees an intricate series of checks and balances within the autonomic nervous system related to body temperature, sleep, heart rate, levels of arousal, and blood pressure.

Structurally, the pituitary is positioned a short distance behind the third-eye center, draping like a testicle from the top of the brain stem. It dwells in its own sanctuary within the sphenoid bone, cradled in a small hollow called the sella turcica, or Turkish Saddle. This cradle has real significance for the subtle body. In Sanskrit, it is poignantly called the *suṣumnā pitham,* the "suṣumnā pedestal." This is where the suṣumnā nāḍī transits through the sphenoid bone as it penetrates the central axis of the body. Notice in figure 7.1 the location of the pituitary gland, just superior to the back portion of the palate. Installed like a jewel in the firmament of the skull, it is buffered by the air pockets of the superior nasopharynx, the sphenoidal sinus, and the fontal sinus.

Called the butterfly bone in Japanese, the sphenoid bone is beautiful, angelic, and otherworldly looking. Its arcing wings soar outward to the lateral skull, and its central sulcus is a nest for the pituitary gland. At the level of the temples, the sphenoid bone spans the skull from side to side (you can palpate the greater wing of the sphenoid just lateral to the outer edge of your eye), and it articulates with every other bone in the head. For this reason the sphenoid is referred to as the keystone of the cranium. In craniosacral mechanics the sphenoid's subtle movements are regularly adjusted by skilled therapists, and when the bone releases, it "floats," thereby inducing states of deep calm.

If you have ever received a sphenoid release, you may recall how deeply relaxing it is. Recipients often slip into a deep sleep that includes periodic still points. In a still point, the pump of cerebrospinal fluid (CSF) is suspended, the entire craniosacral mechanism pauses, and a dynamic stillness pervades the body. This is akin to moments of suspension between inhalation and exhalation, the profound serenity induced in śavāsana and *yoga nidrā*. The still point may be a physiological equivalent to Patañjali's *citta vṛtti nirodha*, the defining verse of the Yoga Sutras that identifies yoga as the suspension of mental activity.

The word for the cerebral chakra, *ājñā*, derives from the Sanskrit *jña*, an archaic term that translates as knowledge or wisdom. Etymologically, this word is akin to the Greek word *gnosis* and is relevant to the strange spelling of the English word *know*. The word *prajñā*, which is the name of our school in Santa Fe, suggests an inherent, embodied wisdom. It is a nonconceptual wisdom, not limited to cognition or intellectual function but likened to a kind of sixth sense. Prajñā is ostensibly the pinnacle of yoga training, a knowledge that comes about through concentrated absorption (*samādhi*).

The ājñā center is a kind of doorway to perception. Perception is always colored by the point of view of the perceiver. Images, thoughts, and memories project on the screen of the mind. They come and go like shadows on the walls of Plato's cave. Thus, the ājñā center in the middle forehead is referred to in traditional Chinese medicine as the Hall of Impressions (*Yintang*). As the name suggests, this is the center where the mind weaves its elaborate brocades.

Related to the third-eye center and the pituitary gland, the sphenoid is the visionary bone of the body. In the subtle body, consciousness is irreducibly linked to light. The pituitary and pineal glands are sensitive to light entering the skull. The pineal gland, located in a pocket behind the brain stem, is a primary site for melatonin biosyn-

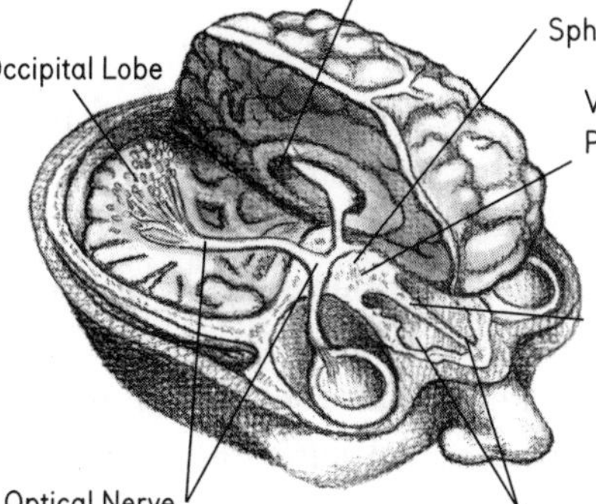

Figure 8.3 The Anatomy of Insight: The Optic Nerve and Sphenoid Bone

thesis and plays a significant role in the body's circadian rhythms. In esoteric anatomy of yoga, the pituitary is associated with sunlight, daytime rhythms, and cycles of activity in the forebrain. The pineal gland is more closely associated with nighttime, the moon, and the back brain.

There are twelve pairs of cranial nerves, and four of the first six are devoted to the eyes. The Optic nerve passes from the eyes through the sphenoid to the occipital lobe at the back of the skull (fig. 8.3). Within the sphenoid bone, the Optic nerve crosses so that half of the visual imprint coming from the right eye passes to the left brain hemisphere, and half of the visual data coming from the left eye passes to the right brain hemisphere. Yogis attributed this neurological weave not only to the eyes but to the two brain hemispheres and vicariously to the entire spine. The braid or plait of the idā, piṅgalā, and suṣumnā nāḍīs has been charted out in many graphic renditions of the chakras (see fig. 7.5).

The fact that the Optic nerve passes from each eyeball to the posterior skull suggests the close association between the hindbrain and vision. In English we have an expression that refers to good intuition and keen sensibility—to have eyes in the back of your head. Along with the third eye in the forehead, it is possible to imagine a fourth eye at the center of the back of the skull (a concept I first learned from Richard Rosen, a yoga teacher in Berkeley, California). In meditation practice, it is valuable to begin with your focus at the third eye in the center of the brow, travel through the sphenoid, and then to a fourth eye at the back of the skull (see fig. 7.2).

PRACTICE

Fourth-Eye Meditation

This visualization begins with relaxing the anatomical eyes, prior to opening the mystical eyes at the center brow and middle back skull. This is a valuable way to release eyestrain and headaches related to eye tension.

Assume a comfortable seated position by supporting your pelvis on a four- to six-inch lift. Begin by drawing the back of your skull gently upward off of your first cervical vertebra while lowering the bridge of your nose. Relax your tongue onto the floor of your mouth. Then dissolve any tension out of your eyes and soften the skin of your upper eyelids. Be sure that your lids do not squeeze or tense against the outer surface of your eyes. Allow your eyelashes to lightly interlace. Widen the sides of your skull so that the outer wings of your sphenoid bone are light and feel as if they are floating. Dilate the skin midway between your eyebrows in the region of the third eye (called *Śiva sṭānam*). According to the *Haṭha Yoga Pradipikā*, expanding the region of the mid-frontal brain allows for an experience of timelessness.

Once your forehead feels open and spacious, concentrate your awareness into your center back skull. As you did at the midpoint of your forehead, visualize widening the skin at the back of your skull, dilating the fourth eye. Sense the visual field within the occipital lobe of your hindbrain expanding. Allow your awareness to be extremely fine, as delicate as the wings of a dragonfly. Sense the ways in which mindful contact with your back skull enables a deeper, more profound state of stillness. Remain for ten to fifteen minutes. Rest in śavāsana afterward for several minutes.

The anatomical eyes allow light into the head through vision. When the mystical third eye opens, the luminosity of clarified consciousness bathes the head with internal light. In Patañjali's Yoga Sutras (III.33), light that pervades the head is equated with visionary power, *mūrdha jyotiṣi siddha darśanam.* A common metaphor for awakening, effulgent light is a sign of revelation. In various invocations to Patañjali, his revelatory form is described as having "one thousand heads of white light" (*sahasra śirasaṃ śvetaṃ*).

Suffusion of light within the skull is associated with rapid shifts in consciousness relating to spiritual transcendence. During the Renaissance in Europe, celestial beings, saints, and angels are surrounded by halos of radiating light. In the subtle body, the suṣumnā, the central column of life, is described as a streak of sunlight, implying that all living beings are derived from the sun and its revelatory light. For this reason, many spin-offs in yoga training involve honorific practices to the sun, like the well-known *sūrya namaskāra* (sun salutation).The body of light is likened not only to sunlight but to other forms of radiance. The celebrated Zen master Hakuin once charged his students to "become a bolt of fine white silk." In a collection called *The Field of Silent Illumination*, the Chinese Zen Master Hongzhi wrote,

> When the stains from old habits are exhausted, the original light appears, blazing through your skull, not admitting any other matters. Vast and spacious, like sky and water merging during autumn, like snow and moon having the same color, this field is without boundary, beyond direction, magnificently one entity without edge or seam.[6]

In the Upaniṣads, luminescence of various kinds is indicative of the state of supreme yoga:

> Fog, smoke, sun, wind, fire, fireflies, lightning, crystals, the moon; these are the preliminary forms which produce the manifestation of *Brahman* in yoga.[7]

This verse from the *Śvetāśvatara Upaniṣad* poetically captures the vibratory nature of light; light that shimmers, sparkles, glistens and gleams as it travels through the nadis of the subtle body. It is living light or manifest light (*prakāśa*) within the fluid-electric matrix of the body. It is identifiable as the pulse of the kundalini that quivers, trembles, and twinkles (*sphuraṇa*) when it flows.

The Living Skull

Only thirty years ago it was commonly believed that the bones of the skull were immobile and inert like the bark of a tree. Yet through research in the fields of osteopathy and craniosacral therapy, it is evident (and palpable) that the cranial bones are perpetually in motion. They "breathe," moving via slight expansive and contractile rhythms following the tidal flow of CSF. The zigzag sutures that interlock the bones are like pieces of a jigsaw puzzle. Unlike the lifeless puzzle, the stretch receptors within the sutures have give, which is particularly important at birth when compressive forces are loaded onto the fetal cranium during delivery.

The cranial bones are constantly in flux, accommodating local pressures within the brain. Even in the course of a day, one can sense changing pressures within the cranium relative to levels of exertion, internal stress, blood pressure, diet, and so on. Cardiovascular changes and neurological shifts regularly impact the synchronistic rhythms of the cranial bones. This is evident when you descend in a jet plane from thirty thousand feet. As the bones of your skull compress, you are prompted to release the pressure by creating an internal yawn. Yawning helps to release the upper end of the throat and pop the auditory tubes. After a flight you may notice how your half-empty plastic water bottle has crumpled and shrunk; it is a distressing thought that the same forces are applied to your skull.

We know that the body as a whole is 80 to 85 percent water, and this applies to the brain and spinal cord that virtually float in clear cerebrospinal fluid. Like an underground spring, the CSF emerges out of a chasm deep in the brain, trickling out from the third ventricle located just above the brain stem. CSF circulates around the cerebral cortex (in Sanskrit called *Śira brahma*), cushioning and protecting it.

On the interior of the skull, the cranial plates are held in place by two intersecting membranes that traverse the skull. In the way that the flesh of a walnut is secured by two paper-thin sheaths, so the brain is moored to the interior of the skull casing by horizontal and verti-

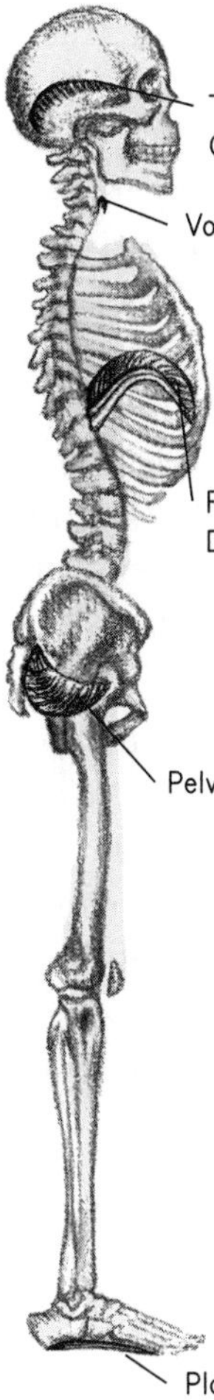

Figure 8.4 Five Diaphragms in Taḍāsana (Mountain Pose)

cal lamina. The vertical sheath, called the falx cerebri, is a sickle-shaped slice of tissue that divides the two hemispheres of the brain. The falx attaches to two internal bony landmarks that correspond to the third eye in front (the crista galli of the ethmoid bone) and the fourth eye in back (the interior occipital protruberance). The horizontal membrane, the tentorium cerebelli, spans the width of the skull, attaches to the inner walls of the temporal bones, and supports the weight of the large forward-thrusting cerebrum. Together the two membranes form a tent-like structure that secures, pads, and surrounds the brain. They provide a fulcrum for movement within the brain, and since they tie into the dural sheathing that encases the spinal cord, they are responsive to movement in the sacrum.

Like all connective tissues in the body, these partitioning membranes change their shape and tension. As a result the brain has room to breathe and pulsate. The tentorium cerebelli is integral to the architecture of the brain since it is a shelf that separates the lower brain (cerebellum) from the higher brain (cerebrum). Like a rooftop on a circus tent, the tentorium is our final horizontal diaphragm in the body (fig. 8.4). The tentorium resonates powerfully with the other horizontal sheaths: the plantar fascia, the perineum, the respiratory diaphragm, and the vocal cord diaphragm. This means that potentially adjustments within the feet or pelvic floor can impact the cranial diaphragm that supports the brain. All of these sheaths distribute forces of strain at key intersections of the body. The tentorium plays a significant role as it is energetically paired with the third-eye center of the skull and is linked structurally to the sphenoid, the pituitary, and the brainstem.

PRACTICE

Feeling Cranial Rhythms

This is a meditative guide to feeling subtle shifts within the bone, connective tissues, and fluid tides of the skull. Assume a comfortable seated position with your pelvis supported on a lift four- to six-inches away from the floor. Begin by settling the bony weight of your sitting bones, legs, and hands. Gently push the crown of your head up toward the ceiling to elongate your neck like a migrating heron. Empty your jaw and allow the skin covering your cheekbones to soften. Let go of any tension in your neck, face, or jaw. Release the skin on the sides of your skull so that your temporal bones feel like they are hovering. This will enable the tentorium, the connective tissue that spans the distance between your temples, to spread. Rest in thoughtless awareness and allow a feeling of serenity to pervade your entire skull. Bring your awareness to the ebb and flow of your breath, and notice any pulses, tremors, tingles, or pressures in and around your skull. Next, bring your awareness to fluid tides within your skull and brain. See if you can sense a slight expansion and contraction of your cranial bones and membranes. Do you feel greater pulsation on the right or left side of your skull? Sense the stretch receptors rhythmically expand and narrow within the zigzag sutures of your interlocking cranial bones. Feel the fluctuations within your brain and sense how it moves ever so slightly, bobbing like seaweed in the waves along the shore. Remain for ten to fifteen minutes.

The Old Brain and New Brain

Homo sapiens (wise humankind) evolved from a four-legged stance to a two-legged stance, a postural shift that freed the hands for toolmaking. As a result, the neocortex ballooned in size. Some evolutionary biologists believe that if it were not for the limitation of the size of the fetal cranium that must pass through the narrow opening of the birth canal, the coils of gray matter within the human frontal brain would have continued to grow exponentially. Within the frontal brain, fifteen to thirty billion neurons pack into a small space and relay high-speed instant messages. The speed of delivery transmitted from cell to cell is lightning fast due in part to a fatty film of myelinated sheathing that wraps around the nerve fibers. Communication within this neural network is rapid fire. Intracranial signals dance across cerebral synapses faster than the information exchange in the nerves outside the skull that rely on biochemical signals. Within the brain, a single axon—which is a miniscule, whiplike hair branching off a neuron—can make up to several thousand synaptic connections with any other neuron. There are one hundred trillion possible neuronal connections within the brain—one thousand times the number of stars in our galaxy. This kind of metacommunication is continuous down the spine, where a thirty-thousand-mile network of nerves relays information from headquarters out to the periphery and from the periphery to the core.[8]

Buried beneath the newest technology of the forebrain is a prehistoric monument. The brain stem consists of the midbrain, the medulla oblongata, and the pons that bridges the right and left hemispheres. This ancient cluster of structures operates below the radar of the cognitive brain. Hardwired to some degree, it oversees basic controls such as temperature, heart rate, hunger, breathing, postural balance, and emotion.

Set deep in the underbelly of the temporal lobes are two jewel-size structures, the amygdalae, which play a significant role in regulating emotion. They are like small flash drives that store both negative and positive memory. In the amygdalae, the sensory stimuli from fear, anger, or desire (saṃskārs) are imprinted and processed. From the amygdala nerve connections relay to the face via the large trigeminal nerve. This suggests why emotions are so often reflected in the face. Because emotions have such a powerful effect on the biorhythms of the subtle body, yoga discipline requires careful processing of the feeling body. Essentially feelings are outside of conscious control and so relate to the instinctual serpent power kuṇḍalinī. It is the hard-drive function of the instinctual brain that haṭha yogis aim to decode and crack, a most complex and arduous task.

The Rise of Consciousness

At the apex of the spinal shaft, rising up into the skull like a sacred edifice, the brain stem is corollary to the kuṇḍalinī, buried in caverns of the lower two chakras. Yogis visualize the brain and spinal cord together as the body of a sinewy snake; not simply a garden-variety snake but the archetypal cobra that possesses a unique ability to rise vertically against gravity from a horizontal position.

The *Śiva liṅga* is a mass of vertical stone whose upward lift, like the primeval rise of the cobra, suggests an essential animating force. Through its verticality the Śiva liṅga—like Stonehenge's monolithic columns—implies the sheer rise of consciousness. The liṅga is a formless phallus that signifies the supreme power of the arch-yogi Śiva. Its rise is a potent reflex necessary to sustain life. The vertical stone of the liṅga stands in a supportive base, the horizontal *yoni,* which is the source for female creative energy and the origin of birth. The alchemical combination of liṅga and yoni not only gives birth to life but suggests how opposing forces are both creative and complementary.

Humankind's upright posture involves a combination of horizontal and vertical planes. We have seen how the five diaphragms support the body in tiers from foot to skull. This horizontality complements the verticality of the spine and brain stem. Like the upward-rising cobra, consciousness stands on end. At the very top of the spinal cord where the cord inserts into the underbelly of the brain (where the brain

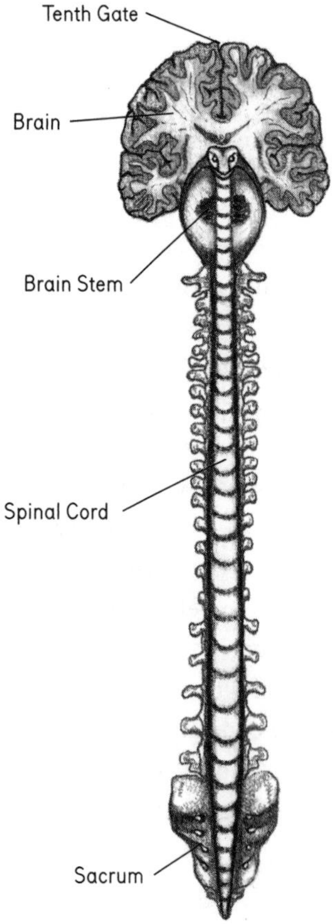

Figure 8.5 Kuṇḍalinī and Brain Stem

rests on the tentorium), the brain stem widens. Akin to the flared hood of the cobra, the brain stem bulges and forms a series of small pouches. This is where the relatively narrow bandwidth of the spinal cord starts to diversify and increase in synaptic complexity as it merges into the brain. In the analogy of the cobra the width of the brain stem mimics the spatial breadth of the cobra's hood, a structure that flares outward when the snake is aroused (fig. 8.5).

Within the brain stem the involuntary nervous system is carefully regulated. All haṭha yoga techniques that involve breath retention, physical poses, fasting, sensory withdrawal, and so on essentially aim to modulate the brain stem's autonomic functioning. As we noted earlier, the kuṇḍalinī force is thought to be latent, coiled up at the opposite end of the spine within the pelvic floor. When the kuṇḍalinī emerges from her lair at the spinal base, she is said to move like a snake through a bamboo tube. In yoga awakening the potency of the kuṇḍalinī is not only a biological event. It is to be accompanied by altruistic motivations such as tolerance, patience, and kindness. According to the *Haṭha Yoga Pradīpikā*, "This energy (*śakti*) is the way to liberation for yogis, and the cause of bondage for the deluded. Whoever knows this knows yoga."[9] The alchemy of raja yoga transforms the raw energy of the reptilian force so that self-protective fear flips into love and divided, obsessive self-consciousness turns into Buddha nature.

The Buddha and the King Cobra

Due to the rigors of yoga practice the expanse of the cobra's hood, rather than a gesture showing malice and vengeance, becomes a symbol of protection. In the parable of Shakyamuni Buddha's prolonged vision quest under the bodhi tree, he was reputed to have meditated for forty days and nights before attaining enlightenment. While meditating he was assaulted by nefarious forces. The demon of temptation and self-reification (*Mara*) threatened to rattle his concentration. As the story goes, his psychological turbulence was matched by terrific climactic shifts: wind and rain from a sudden, unseasonal tempest came overhead. In the midst of this threat, a king cobra stood upright behind the

Buddha-to-be and provided shelter. Paradoxically, the serpent's protective hood and seven heads (perhaps one for each chakra) enabled the Buddha to abandon any impulses meant to defend, qualify, or perpetuate his individual personality. It was in part due to this shelter that the Buddha was able to attain great awakening, suggesting that the reptilian force is an integral component, if not a necessary alliance, in the process of awakening.

The Thousand-Petaled Lotus

The sahasrāra chakra, the seventh chakra at the crown of the head, is described as a thousand-petaled lotus. Like the mention of ten thousand things in Taoism and Zen, *sahasrāra* implies an infinite number. Thus, the crown chakra is vast like a boundless sky, void of name, form, or personality. Space and sky are analogies for a boundless mind as we have already seen. For this reason, the crown chakra is also known as the *śūnya cakra*, the chakra of boundlessness or emptiness. The thousand-petalled lotus is a metaphor for the innumerable connections possible within the brain. In visual renderings of the crown chakra, the entire Sanskrit alphabet is inscribed onto the multipetaled lotus, suggesting that all sound and language emerge from space and silence. The cranial bloom stands for the totality of sound and silence.

Classical texts devoted to the chakras such as the Ṣaṭ Chakra Nirūpaṇa describe the thousand petals of the flower as turned downward prior to awakening. As an analogy for enlightenment, they

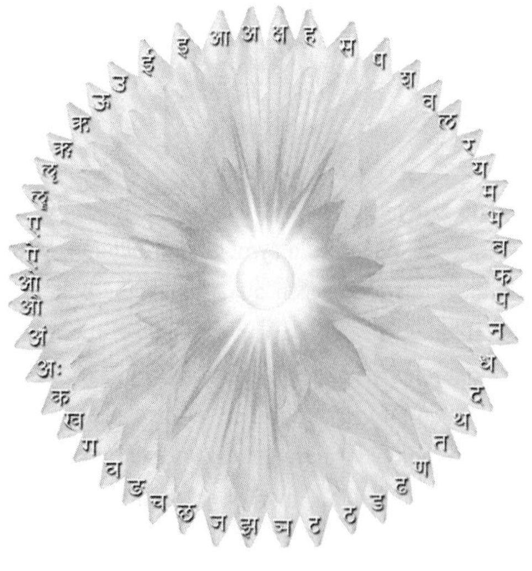

Figure 8.6 The Thousand-Petal Lotus

blossom and turn upward. In today's scientific parlance, this bloom suggests opening of new neural pathways within the brain and central nervous system. Brain plasticity is critical to health and to leading a life without strong bias and prejudice. Thomas Merton, a Trappist monk, Zen student, author, and social activist, prolific in the 1950s and 1960s, referred to this plasticity as a "space of liberty." In *The Other Side of the Mountain*, he wrote:

> The contemplative life must provide an area, a space of liberty, of silence, in which possibilities are allowed to surface and new choices "beyond routine choices" become manifest. It should create a new experience of time, not as a stopgap, stillness, but as "temps vierge," not a blank to be filled or an untouched space to be conquered or violated, but a space which can enjoy its own potentialities and hopes; and its own presence to itself. One's own time. But not dominated by ego and its demands. Hence open to others—compassionate time.[10]

Merton's "space of liberty," the untouched space that enjoys its own potential outside of habitual thought and behavior, is not something otherworldly but available by way of a spacious and open mind. The name of the sahasrāra chakra could be Boundless Awareness, or as it is said in Zen, Big Mind. The metaphor of the cranial bloom suggests a move toward an all-inclusive awareness that is open, continuously, to the new.

The Jewel in the Lotus

A further elaboration on the lotus within the skull involves a jewel of a most unusual kind. The jewel (*mani*) is installed in the central plexus of the brain. Its surface is exquisitely wrought, inconceivable by design, and its mirror-like nature infinitely reflects the things of the world. Unlike a mirror, this jewel is also equipped with boundless generative potential. Like the liquid cortex of the earth, we can imagine this jewel to be dynamic and ever changing. Paradoxically, while changeable, the jewel is diamond-like, adamantine, and indestructible. It cannot be splintered or fragmented, reduced or augmented in any way. Thus, it is constant, singular, and enduring and has been since the beginning of time.

The metaphor of the mind-jewel appears significantly in Vajrayāna schools of Tibetan Buddhism. *Vajra* means jewel or diamond (it also can mean lightning), and *āyana* refers to a vehicle or path. Thus *Vajrayāna* is the Way of the Diamond. As an analogy for the unitive state of mind in meditation, the diamond stands for the unbreakable nature of mind. Like the discriminating sword of wisdom, this mind-jewel has the capacity to cut through all things, including the sticky cobwebs of delusive thought. By necessity, the diamond mind too cuts off any edifying notions of itself.

The most well-known and often repeated prayer throughout Tibetan Buddhist practice is the six-syllable mantra *om maṇi padme hum,* translated as "homage to *maṇi* the jewel in the lotus (*padma*)." The power of this mantra generates compassion and unbreakable equanimity. And so the water flower of the brain cradles a jewel of infinite wisdom and kindness in its pithy core.

The Top of the Skull

We now turn to the vital structures at the apex of the skull. At birth, two apertures in the top of the skull are not yet fused—the anterior and posterior fontanels. These "little fountains" accommodate the growth and expansion of the brain, and allow the fetal cranium to compress during delivery. Compressive forces applied to an infant's skull during passage through the birth canal are critical to help jump-start the craniosacral rhythm, and babies who are delivered via C-section may lack the coherence and positive amplitude needed for healthy motility of the cranial sutures. Postpartum, the gap in the anterior fontanel remains open for approximately two years. This soft spot on an infant has a spongy consistency, like a ripe plum. At the opening of this fontanel it is possible to feel the arterial pulse of a newborn's heart. That the pulse of the heart can be felt at the top skull suggests the rhythmic accord between heart rate and the brain.

Earlier in this chapter, we noted nine gates or apertures in the body that allow passage between the interior self and the external environment. The anterior fontanel at the crown of the head is identified as the *tenth gate* and a primary path for the suṣumnā nāḍī and the kuṇḍalinī (see fig. 8.5). The anterior fontanel, also called the bregma, is formed by the intersection of the coronal and sagittal sutures. In the mystical traditions, it is the primary opening to the central channel, the pathway of *prāna,* and is the spot where the soul enters the body at the time of birth and departs at the time of death. For this reason, the anterior fontanel is identified as *Brāhma randhra,* or the "Aperture of Brāhma," and in subtle-body awakening, passage through this aperature leads to an experience of supreme delight (*brāhmānanda*).

The Skull Cap

The cup-shaped crown of the head is charged with vitality. Shaped like a singing bowl, the roof of the cranium, called the *kapāla*, circumscribes the life force that resides inside the orb of the skull. The prefix of the word *kapāla, ka,* means time, and *pāla* means ruler or governor. Thus, the skullcap, the lid of the body, symbolically binds human existence to the world of time. The forehead and forebrain are linked to time-bound plans, projects, and to-do lists. In Āyurveda the *kapāla marma* is located on the forehead at the level of the hairline just above the third-eye center.

Some sects of Hindu and Buddhist Tantra use the skullcap as a ritual implement. The cup-shaped upper cranium serves either as a begging bowl for wandering ascetics or as an implement for making offerings to local deities. By taking food from the kapāla begging bowl, the yogi is reminded of the constraints of this time-bound world (eating is an essential worldly act) while in "left-hand" (taboo) Tantric paths, drinking blood or wine from the kapāla is thought to be a means to transcend the body and time.

The Hundred Meeting Place

From the anterior fontanel, we move to the very top of the skull, the polestar of the entire body, called the "overlord point" in Āyurveda (*adhipati marma*). This is approximately the point that bears the weight of the body during headstand. Thus śīrṣāsana is referred to as the "king of all the poses" and is a direct means to access the central channel. The overlord point is located on the sagittal suture, the uppermost cranial seam. The sagittal suture orients with the central axis of the body, including the midline between the two brain hemispheres and the midline of the palate. It aligns with the midpoints of the five diaphragms: the mid-tentorium, the gap between the vocal cords, the central tendon of the diaphragm, the central tendon of the perineum, and the center sole of the foot. Like mystic ley lines that are purported to orient geological landmarks on the earth's surface, the sagittal suture coordinates with the sacred central channel, the suṣumnā.

In traditional Chinese medicine the summit of the crown chakra is called the Hundred Meeting Place (*Du 20*). It is the highest acupressure point in the body located along the Governing Vessel, which begins at the tip of the coccyx (see fig. 2.8). In the way that the North Pole is the convergence site for the longitudinal global meridians, the center point of the skullcap is where all yang meridians in the body unite. In qigong practice this is a point where we absorb the "energy of heaven" and draw it down into the body.

PRACTICE

Meditation on the Crown Chakra

This meditation helps bring sensitivity to the three main marma points on the top of the skull: the *Brahma randhra, Adhipati marma,* and *Śiva randhra.* Collectively these points help to reduce vāta imbalance (emotional disturbance), reduce tension headaches and intracranial pressure, and promote circulation through the brain.

Assume a comfortable seated pose so that your spine can lengthen upward without strain. Balance your skull so that it is not tipping right or left or pitching forward or backward. Place the tip of your middle fingers at the top of the helix of each ear and trace a line to the uppermost pole of your skull. This is the apex of your body, the One Hundred Meeting Point. Using one middle-finger pad, place light pressure on this point for several minutes in order to bring heightened sensitivity to your crown. When you release contact, observe any light pulsation at this point, the Adhipati marma.

Next, rest the heel of your hand on the middle of your forehead and extend your palm upward toward the top of your skull. Where your middle finger now rests is close to the anterior fontanel. Apply soft, steady pressure with your finger pad here for several minutes, then release. This is the Brāhma randhra marma point.

Come to the apex of your head once more, then slide backward two inches to the place on the back of your skull where the slope begins to turn down. Apply light pressure on this point, the approximate location of the posterior fontanel. Release and notice any pulsation at the back edge of your crown. This is the Śiva randhra marma point (see fig. 7.2).

Now press all three points simultaneously and hold for several minutes. Afterward, rest your hands and sense any heat or strain evaporating from the top of your skull.

Imagine the top of your skull to be porous. Visualize it opening to the sky. Imagine a bath of light pouring like an oblation through the top of your head, bathing all the structures of your skull and brain. Visualize this light bath seeping down your neck, through your chest and abdomen, and pooling in your reproductive organs. Imagine the way this internal bath of light soothes all your tissues, including nerves, organs, and glands. Take time to soak any structure in your body that may need healing. Stay for ten minutes or more. Afterward, rest in śavāsana for several minutes.

Śiva's Moon

As the crown flower of innumerable petals opens its radiance, it emits a cool glowing light. The Ṣaṭ Cakra Nirūpaṇa, likely composed in the mid-sixteenth century and the most comprehensive collection of sutras on the chakra system, compares the radiance of the uppermost skull to the moon: "Within [the *sahasrāra chakra*] is a full, clear, and pure moon, without any marks. Its liquid moonlight spreads a cool profusion of supreme essence."[11] In keeping with the glacial environs of the polar cap, the sheen of the top calvarium is characterized not by intense heat but by a cool lunar glow.

Śiva has the ultimate cool demeanor, unfazed by the activity of the world, as captured by Kālidāsa, the greatest of all Sanskrit poets, in the tale *The Origin of the Young God* (*Kumārasambhava*). At the outset of the story, Śiva is deep in yogic concentration, perched high atop a glacial crevasse in the Himalayan plateau. The environment is contiguous with his samādhi: cool, remote, and unbreakable. (However, numerous glaciers of the Himalayas have been melting due to global warming, evidence that not only the ice caps but the life-sustaining reserve of Śiva's meditative power may be disappearing.) Like the vast expanse of glacier around him, Śiva is immobile, his prāṇa withheld. His serene, unflappable samādhi provides the necessary counterpoint for a world gone mad with activity.

Śiva sits in padmāsana (lotus pose), his gaze fixed on the ājñā chakra (his third eye), and his mass of hair, the symbol of his extraordinary life-force and longevity, is coiled *(jaṭa)* on top of his head. The magnitude of his jaṭa is so great that he requires the sturdiest of hair clips to keep it in place. So Śiva secures his pile of dreadlocks with the decorative and fluorescent sliver moon (*chandra*). The moon is the most appropriate heavenly body to match Śiva's imperturbable calm. The moon emanates tranquillity (sattva) and yogic samādhi, and has a radiant watery glow. Unlike the sun whose light offers sharp contrast to the things of the world, the moon's luminosity is diffuse, soft, and dreamy. Within the cranium, the foreskull is associated with the sun and the world of form, while the back skull is correlated with the moon and states of reflection, contemplation, and quietude.

Inside the cranium is the lesser-known lunar chakra, called the *soma chakra,* enshrined in the back of the skull. Soma is associated with the incandescent moon and the light-synthesizing function of the pineal gland. Aligned to the tides of the ocean, the fluid tide of CSF, the underworld of dreams, and the divine feminine, the lunar chakra is a realm where there is no fixity. Shaṇkarācarya, the celebrated philosopher of *advaita vedānta* (teachings on nondualism), describes the perfuse radiance of the moon as a source of ongoing rejuvenation:

> I extol bhavānī whose body is nectar and whose very form is joy. She triumphantly shines forth at the end of a string of six lotuses. Exceedingly lustrous in the middle way of the suṣumnā, she melts the moon of nectar to drink its light.[12]

In yoga meditation, awareness is deliberately drawn away from the frontal lobes of the brain and guided to the back brain. In the back brain the moon is the abode of introspective, lucid, mirror-like awareness. Divinely intoxicating, the lunar glow of meditative awareness has a nourishing and cooling effect on the entire body. Inclusive of all transitions through her phases, the moon is a continuous reminder of flux; passing from emptiness to fullness and contraction to expansion, the immortal moon, like the light of consciousness, is enduring.

Notes

Foreword

1. Translation by Richard Freeman.

Introduction

1. Ken Kesey, "Ken Kesey, The Art of Fiction No. 136," *The Paris Review* (Spring 1994): www.theparisreview.org/interviews/1830/the-art-of-fiction-no-136-ken-kesey.

Chapter 1

1. Nicolai Bachman, Aṣṭāṅga Yoga Mantra, 2014.
2. C. G. Jung, *The Psychology of Kuṇḍalinī Yoga* (Princeton, NJ: Princeton University Press, 1996), 30.
3. The five elements (*pancha tattvas*) and their chakras:

Sense	**Anatomy**	**Element**	**Chakra**
Olfactory	Nostrils	Earth (*pṛthivī*)	*Mūlādhāra*
Gustatory	Tongue	Water (*āp*)	*Svādhiṣthāna*
Visual	Eyes	Fire (*tejas*)	*Maṇipūra*
Tactile	Skin	Air (*vāyu*)	*Anāhāta/Viśuddha*
Auditory	Ears	Space (*ākāśa*)	*Ājñā/Sahasrāra*

4. Nicolai Bachman and Tias Little, Taittirīya Upaniṣad, ch. 2, verse 1 (2014).
5. Moshe Feldenkrais, *Body and Mature Behavior: A Study of Anxiety, Sex, Gravitation, and Learning* (Madison, CT: International Universities Press, 1992), 70.
6. Kazuaki Tanahashi, *Moon in a Dewdrop* (New York: North Point Press, Farrar, Straus and Giroux, 1985), 99–101.
7. The complete Aṣṭāṅga Yoga Invocation:

   vande gurūṇāṃ caraṇāravinde
   saṃsarśita-svātma-sukhāvabodhe
   niḥśreyase jāṅgalikāyamāne
   saṃāra-hālāhala-moha-śāntyai.
   ābāhu puruṣākāraṃ
   śaṅkha-cakrāsi-dhāriṇaṃ
   sahasra-śirasaṃ śvetaṃ
   praṇamāmi Patañjalim.

   I honor the lotus feet of all the gurus,
   which awaken and manifest joy in oneself;
   beyond comparison, appearing as a snake-charmer (śiva)
   for pacifying the poisonous delusion of saṃsāra (the cycle of birth and death).
   In the form of a man up to the shoulders,
   holding the conch (divine sound), discus (wheel of time)
   and sword (discrimination),
   thousand-headed, white,
   I bow respectfully to Patañjali.
8. "Back Pain Stats," *American Spinal Decompression Association*: www.americanspinal.com/back-pain-stats.html.
9. The following are the six diaphragms and their associated bandhas: feet-plantar fascia/pada bandha; pelvic floor/*mūla* bandha; respiratory diaphragm/uḍḍīyāna bandha; vocal cords/*jālandhara banda*; palate/jihvhabandha, khechari mudra; and tentorium cerebelli/shambhavi mudra.
10. Peter Deadman, Mazin Al-Khafaji, and Kevin Baker, *A Manual of*

Acupuncture (East Sussex England: Journal of Chinese Medicine Publications, 2007), 337.

11. Martin Palmer, *The Book of Chuang Tzu* (London: Penguin, Arkana, 1996), 47.
12. Peter Deadman, Mazin Al-Khafaji, and Kevin Baker, *A Manual of Acupuncture* (East Sussex England: Journal of Chinese Medicine Publications, 2007), 30.

Chapter 2

1. T. S. Eliot, *Four Quartets* (New York: Harcourt, Brace and World Inc., 1971), 59. Used by permission.
2. Janet Travell and David Simons, *Myofascial Pain and Dysfunction Volume II, The Trigger Point Manual* (New York: Williams and Wilkins, 1983), 192.
3. Srisa Chandra Vasu and Rai Bahadur, *The Śiva Saṁhitā* (New Delhi, India: Munshiram Manoharlal, 1999), 62.
4. Nicolai Bachman and Tias Little, *The Bhagavad Gita* (unpublished translation, 2014).
5. Aṣṭāṅga Yoga (Eight Limbs of Yoga):
    1. yama: social ethics, "restraints"
    2. niyama: personal ethics, internal restraints
    3. āsana: posture, sitting
    4. prāṇāyāma: breath regulation
    5. pratyāhāra: internalization of the senses, "drawing back"
    6. dhāraṇā: focus, concentration
    7. dhyāna: maintaining a focus, meditation
    8. samādhi: complete absorbtion

Chapter 3

1. Kaz Tanahashi and Allan Baillie, *Lotus* (Somerville, MA: Wisdom Publications, 2006), 48. Used by permission.
2. A. L. Rosatelli, A. M. Agur, and S. Chhaya, "The Anatomy of the Interosseous Region of the Sacroiliac Joint," *The Journal of Orthopaedic and Sports Physical Therapy* 36 (4) (April 2006): 200–8, www.ncbi.nlm.nih.gov/pubmed/16676869.

Chapter 4

1. Norman O. Brown, *Love's Body* (New York: Vintage Books, 1966), 183.
2. Nicolai Bachman and Tias Little, *The Bhagavad Gita* (unpublished translation, 2014).
3. M.V. Kamath, *Gandhi: A Spiritual Journey* (Mumbai: Indus Source-Books, 2007), 97.
4. Nicolai Bachman and Tias Little, *The Bhagavad Gita* (unpublished translation, 2014).
5. Nicolai Bachman and Tias Little, *The Haṭha Yoga Pradipika,* ch. 3, verses 55–56.
6. S. Radhakrishnan, *The Principal Upanishads* (Amherst, NY: Humanity Books, 1992), 456.
7. Jean-Pierre Barral, *Visceral Manipulation II* (Seattle, WA: Eastland Press, 1989), 99.
8. Ibid., 99.
9. S. Radhakrishnan, *The Principal Upanishads* (Amherst, NY: Humanity Books, 1992), 558.
10. In this verse from the *Aṣṭāṅga Hrdayam, rasa* is the progenitor of the seven bodily *dhātus* (tissues):
    Rasad raktam, tato mamsam, mamsan medas, tato 'sthi ca I
    Asthno majja, tatah shukram, sukrad garbhah prajayate II

    From chyme comes blood, from that muscle (or flesh),
    from muscle fat, from that bone
    From bone marrow, from that semen, from semen is born the fetus
11. Michael D. Gershon, *The Second Brain* (New York: Harper Perennial, 1998).

Chapter 5

1. Shunryu Suzuki, *Zen Mind, Beginner's Mind* (New York: Weatherhill Inc., 1970), 29.
2. S. Radhakrishnan, *The Principal Upanishads* (Amherst, NY: Humanity Books, 1992), 549.

3. Ibid., 554.
4. Tulku Urgyen, *Rainbow Painting* (Kathmandu, Nepal: Rangjung Yeshe Publications, 1995), 90.

Chapter 6

1. Kaz Tanahashi and Allan Baillie, *Lotus* (Somerville, MA: Wisdom Publications, 2006), 16. Used by permission.
2. Lama Mipham, *Calm and Clear* (Berkeley, CA: Dharma Publishing, 1973), 46. Used by permission.
3. Alexander Tsiaras, *The Architecture and Design of Man and Woman* (New York: Doubleday, 2004), 168.
4. Jan Gonda, *The Vision of the Vedic Poets* (The Hague: Mouton and Co., 1963), 276.
5. Nicolai Bachman and Tias Little, *The Katha Upanisad,* ch. 6, verse 17 (unpublished translation, 2014).
6. Peter Deadman, Mazin Al-Khafaji, and Kevin Baker, *A Manual of Acupuncture* (East Sussex, England: Journal of Chinese Medicine Publications, 2007), 375.
7. Nicolai Bachman and Tias Little, *The Katha Upanisad,* ch. 6, verse 15 (unpublished translation 2014).
8. Nicolai Bachman and Tias Little, *The Bhagavad Gita* (unpublished translation, 2014).
9. Nicolai Bachman and Tias Little, *The Vijnana-bhairava,* verse 49 (unpublished translation, 2014).
10. Valerie Roebuck, *The Upanishads* (New York: Penguin Books, 2003), 284.

Chapter 7

1. Roberto Calasso, *Ka: Stories of the Mind and Gods of India* (New York: Alfred Knopf Inc., 1998), 234.
2. Swami Muktibodhananda, *Haṭha Yoga Pradipika* (Bihar, India: Bihar School of Yoga, 1985), 206.
3. Peter Deadman, Mazin Al-Khafaji, and Kevin Baker, "A Manual of Acupuncture," *Journal of Chinese Medicine Publications* (2007): 549.

4. Herman Hesse, *Siddhartha* (New York: New Directions, 1951), 122.
5. Nicolai Bachman and Tias Little, *Maitri Upanisad,* ch. 6, verse 21, 2014.

Chapter 8

1. Red Pine, *The Zen Teachings of Bodhidharma* (New York: North Point Press, 1987), 21.
2. Nicolai Bachman and Tias Little, *The Bhagavad Gita* (unpublished translation, 2014).
3. Hugh Milne, *The Heart of Listening, Volume* 2 (Berkeley, CA: North Atlantic Books, 1995), 190.
4. Thomas Hanna, *Somatics* (Cambridge, MA: Da Capo Press, 1988), 50–51.
5. Keith Dowman, *The Flight of the Garuda* (Somerville, MA: Wisdom Publications, 2003), 76. Used by permission.
6. Taigen Daniel Leighton and Yi Wu, *Cultivating the Empty Field: The Silent Illumination of Zen Master Hongzhi* (San Francisco: North Point Press, 1991), 8–9.
7. S. Radhakrishnan, *The Principal Upanishads* (Amherst, NY: Humanity Books, 1992), 721.
8. Alexander Tsiaras, *The Architecture and Design of Man and Woman* (New York: Doubleday, 2004), 49.
9. Nicolai Bachman and Tias Little, *The Haṭha Yoga Pradipika,* ch. 3, verse 107 (unpublished translation, 2014).
10. Thomas Merton, *The Other Side of the Mountain: The End of the Journey* (New York: Harper Collins, 1998), 262.
11. Nicolai Bachman and Tias Little, *Ṣaṭ Cakra Nirūpaṇa* (unpublished translation, 2014).
12. Richard Freeman, Bhavani Bhujangam, verse 1 (unpublished translation, 2014).

Afterword

At the end of this long pilgrimage through the rich interior of the body, it is clear that we have only begun to plumb the depths of this vast subject. Queries continue to linger as they should: What is prāṇa? And what is really meant by yoga? That is, what should the daily practitioner, through her practice rituals, yoke herself to? In the yoga lab, working with the body and mind, it is good to keep these inquires alive. This book proposes that it is possible, by reconnaissance of a most delicate kind, to explore the subtle body right at the sublime edge of sensation and perception. This is the edge where matter turns to pure spirit, and the body-mind goes through an alchemical change impossible to put into language. It involves a kind of metamorphosis, like the cicada that sheds its exoskeleton at the end of its life span. The confines of a limited, individualized self are dropped and something else emerges, something tender, vulnerable, and more open. The journey through the subtle body—through layers and layers of connective tissue, synapse, and cell—includes divestiture of something completely and utterly intangible. This is the rub, for the self truly has no form. The self for all its character and color, so central to what we have been calling the subtle body, is not solid after all. It is more like mist or vapor or, to use the old adage of the Buddha, like a bubble on a fast-moving stream.

The great exfoliation of self requires a movement on the vertical axis—down into the depths and upward toward sky. Stranded on the horizontal axis, one is likely to remain attached to the character-role, the microcosm of self that we live through socially and in seclusion. Movement on the vertical axis, down into the realm of the underworld or upward to the heavens, allows for connection to a vast, fluid, and timeless realm. Although we have been partial to ascension in this book, the move is equally down into the depth of the psyche. The depths include the realm of myth, the unconscious, the involuntary nervous system, and the kuṇḍalinī. It is always and forever outside the grasp of control.

I hope that all readers of this book and practitioners at large take the plunge into this fertile, elusive, and strange realm. Any rupture of the husk of personality may not be so subtle after all. Yet I find it is best to proceed breath by breath, sensation by sensation through the various strata of the enveloping shell. This has been our journey through the subtle body. May all beings have the fortitude, the perseverance, and the loving guidance to make this breakthrough.

—Tias Little, Santa Fe, New Mexico, July 2014

Acknowledgments

I would like to thank a number of people who have helped make this book possible. First and foremost my editor at Shambhala, Rochelle Bourgault, who helped me keep focus throughout the project. My colleague, dearest friend, and Sanskrit guru Nicolai Bachman who collaborated with me to translate many of the Sanskrit verses in this book, reviewed all Sanskrit transliterations, and was my advisor on a number of historical yoga references (www.sanskritsounds.com). His generosity is boundless. Also I would like to thank Richard Rosen for his ongoing encouragement, support, and insightful teachings. I wish to acknowledge the loquacious Richard Freeman as one of my very first yoga mentors and for his real kindness in providing the preface.

I am very grateful for Marisol Baird's creative hand and astute design sense as chief illustrator on this project (www.marisolbaird.com). May her career flower in many wonderful ways. I would like to thank Anne Hart for her careful reading of the manuscript and fine suggestions. I would also like to thank my older brother William for his advice and guidance in helping shape this book. I offer many thanks to Ruth Hulett for her advice and guidance on the theory and practice of traditional Chinese medicine. I am grateful for Linda Spackman's insights on prenatal yoga. I would like to thank Dr. Premal Khetia for his insightful points on the throat chakra. I am grateful to both Nicolai Bachman and Todd Bush for allowing me to include their chakra art in this manuscript. I owe many thanks to my staff: Holly Porter, for her ongoing support, and to B. Milder for her careful eye in editing the manuscript. I would also like to thank Janine Pearson for her contribution to codifying the artwork in this book.

I would like to extend much love and gratitude to my dedicated and loving wife, Sūrya, for her ongoing support and providing me the opportunity to offer my teachings to the world. Her dedication to the yoga path and profound knowledge of the subtle body are inspiring in her own right. She created many fine meals and brewed many pots of oolong tea for me throughout the long process of writing this book.

Last, I would like to thank the many teachers who have inspired and guided me over my thirty years of practice and study. This includes my anatomy and bodywork instructors, my āsana teachers, and my meditation guides. All that I share in this book stems from the brilliant instruction I have received from others.

References

Bainbridge Cohen, Bonnie. *Sensing, Feeling and Action.* Northampton, MA: Contact Editions, 1993.

Becker, Rollin. *Life in Motion.* Portland, OR: Stillness Press, 1997.

Deadman, Peter. *A Manual of Acupuncture.* East Sussex, UK: Journal of Chinese Medicine Publications, 2007.

Hanna, Thomas. *Somatics.* Cambridge, MA: Da Capo Press, 1988.

Juhan, Deane. *Job's Body.* Barrytown, NY: Station Hill Press, 1987.

Kaptchuk, Ted. *The Web That Has No Weaver.* Chicago: Congdon and Weed, 1983.

Levine, Peter. *Waking the Tiger.* Berkeley, CA: North Atlantic Books, 1997.

Milne, Hugh. *The Heart of Listening.* Berkeley, CA: North Atlantic Books, 1996.

Muktibodhananda. *Hatha Yoga Pradipika.* Varanasi, India: Swami Satyasangananda Saraswati, 1985.

Muller-Ortega, Paul. *The Triadic Heart of Siva.* Albany: SUNY Press, 1989.

Myers, Tom. *Anatomy Trains.* London: Churchill Livingstone, 2001.

Netter, Frank. *Atlas of Human Anatomy.* Philadelphia: Saunders, 2006.

Radhakrishnan, S. *The Principal Upanishads.* Amherst, NY: Humanity Books, 1992.

Rolf, Ida. *Rolfing: The Integration of Human Structures.* New York: Harper and Row, 1977.

Shultz, Louis, and Rosemary Feitis. *The Endless Web.* Berkeley, CA: North Atlantic Books, 1996.

Singh, Jaideva. *The Yoga of Delight, Wonder and Astonishment.* Albany: SUNY Press, 1991.

Sumner, Ged, and Steve Haines. *Cranial Intelligence.* London: Singing Dragon, 2010.

Suzuki, Shunryu. *Zen Mind/Beginner's Mind.* New York: Weatherhill, 1970.

Travell, Janet, and David Simons. *Myofascial Pain and Dysfunction: The Trigger Point Manuals.* Baltimore: Williams and Wilkins, 1983.

Tsiaras, Alexander. *The Architecture and Design of Man and Woman.* New York: Doubleday, 2004

Upledger, John, and Jon Vredevoogd. *Cranial-Sacral Therapy.* Seattle: Eastland Press, 1983.

Zimmer, Heinrich. *Myths and Symbols in Indian Art and Civilization.* Washington, DC: Bollingen Foundation, 1946.

Index of Guided Practices

Index

Pages in italics represent figures.